THE BLUE CROSS
& BLUE SHIELD GUIDE TO
Staying Well

Contemporary Books, Inc.
Chicago

Editorial director: Duane R. Carlson, vice-president, Communications, Blue Cross and Blue Shield Associations

Text illustrations: Sam Thiewes
Text layout: Jan Roy

Copyright © 1982 by the Blue Cross and Blue Shield Associations
All rights reserved
Published by Contemporary Books, Inc.
180 North Michigan Avenue, Chicago, Illinois 60601
Manufactured in the United States of America
Library of Congress Catalog Card Number: 81-71076
International Standard Book Number: 0-8092-5717-3 (cloth)
                                                           0-8092-5716-5 (paper)

Published simultaneously in Canada by
Beaverbooks, Ltd.
150 Lesmill Road
Don Mills, Ontario M3B 2T5
Canada

Contents

CONTRIBUTORS

The text of this book was prepared under the supervision of the faculty of The Life Management Group, La Jolla, California, represented by:

Howard F. Hunt, Ph.D., president of The Life Management Group and chairman of the department of physical education, University of California, San Diego

Daniel T. Brumfield, M.D., psychiatrist in private practice, Del Mar, California, and lecturer in the extension division, University of California, San Diego

Gary J. Frost, Ph.D., behavioral psychologist and manager of corporate training and development, Cubic Corporation, San Diego, California

Robyn Hunt, M.F.A., member of the faculty and lecturer, University of California, San Diego

Vicky Newman, M.S., R.D., staff nutritionist, University of California Hospital, San Diego, and lecturer at the medical school and hospital, University of California, San Diego

E. Lee Rice, D.O., physician in private practice, San Diego, and medical director of the San Diego Sports Medicine Center

CONSULTANTS

Phillips L. Gausewitz, M.D., director of the health and fitness program, Scripps Memorial Hospitals, La Jolla, California

Kenneth Smyth, M.D., medical director of the Idaho Elks Rehabilitation Hospital, Boise, Idaho

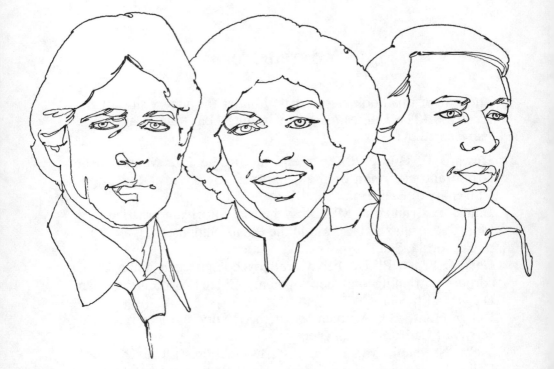

1

Wellness

Nothing in life is as precious or can give you as much pleasure as good health. Yet, few qualities can be as inexpensively attained or universally available.

Wellness—which is a combination of physical fitness and sound mental health—is your birthright. But chances are good that over the years you may have squandered much of it by neglecting to follow good health practices.

Lifestyle is a popular word these days. And while it's often carelessly used, for our purposes lifestyle is simply the way you live—the things you do that affect your health.

Something as important and desirable as wellness would seem to be priceless. Yet, most of us have spent a great deal of our lives with habits that can damage or destroy our physical well-being and mental health.

A lifestyle that encompasses sound health and outstanding physical and mental fitness costs little to maintain, it can't be stolen from you or taxed, it's enjoyable almost from the first moment you accept and start practicing it, and it is well within your grasp.

A healthy lifestyle not only will add to the length of your life (your life span), but also will improve the quality of life, the richness and simple joy of being alive.

Living longer—and living fit—allows you thousands more hours of vibrant and active living, a wider range of activity, and the opportunity for greater accomplishment. Living better can also mean living in greater physical comfort, ease, and enjoyment in carrying out your daily tasks. It will allow you to experience life with added strength, vitality, creativity, and pleasure.

If you are generally healthy, you should integrate three basic factors into your life in order to enjoy better health. These are proper nutrition, regular exercise, and efficient stress management. The manner and consistency with which you perform this integration procedure will ultimately dictate the quality of your lifestyle.

In the pages that follow, you will learn not only that you can and should take responsibility for your wellness, but that it's easy and can be fun.

In Chapter 2 you will discover how to properly nourish your body with health-promoting foods. Chapter 3 will teach you how to exercise your muscles and cardiorespiratory system regularly and in a way that suits your tastes and fits your schedule. In Chapter 4 you will learn how to recognize and eliminate situations that would cause stress and damage both your physical and emotional health. And, by eliminating or reducing stress, you can greatly improve your health and fitness lifestyle. The book's final Chapter 5 will teach you how to change your bad habits into good ones and to integrate nutrition, exercise, and stress reduction into a workable personal lifestyle.

No one will force you to adopt any of the health and fitness practices described in this book. You must make the decision to do this for yourself. You needn't have the iron-willed determination of a professional athlete; you can proceed at your own pace and enjoy the positive changes in your health and fitness lifestyle.

Above all, achieving good health and fitness should be an *en-*

joyable process. You can do as much or as little as you like toward making the changes in your life suggested here, as long as you enjoy the process. You can proceed as slowly or as quickly as you find comfortable and enjoyable. And remember that even small positive changes in your lifestyle can increase the length and improve the quality of your life.

An unhealthful lifestyle can be directly responsible for many of our health problems today, such as obesity, stress, physical inactivity, hypertension, abuse of drugs, alcohol, and tobacco, dietary excesses, diabetes, depression, insomnia, stroke, heart attack, frequent flu and colds, and general unhappiness.

Given that many of these physical and mental ills and conditions are often the result of maintaining an unhealthful lifestyle, it's essential to realize that most of them are preventable—either totally or to a great degree—simply by making intelligent and health-promoting modifications to your current lifestyle. These modifications are not painful, complicated processes of giving up your present lifestyle to accept a radical, somewhat lonely new one. They mean eating nourishing and health-promoting food, exercising vigorously, and responding effectively and easily to changes and stressful situations. So doesn't it make sense to decide to adopt a new health-and-fitness lifestyle?

In the pages that follow, you will find the Life Management Self-Evaluation Test, which shows you how to find out for yourself what your own "health score" is now. Take the test by answering all the questions, then adding or subtracting the number of points indicated in each question or part, to get your total score.

As you finish Chapters 2, 3, 4, and 5, you'll find the portion of the Life Management Test that applies to each chapter. Think about how—over the next year—you can improve your first score using the knowledge you've gained from reading this book. Then take each part of the test again, after completing each chapter, with the determination to set a new health goal for yourself. How much do you think you can improve? Can you cut down or give up smoking? Eat fewer sweets and fats? Exercise some every day? Avoid stressful quarrels at home and hassles at work? What? Be realistic. Don't put down goals you know you won't be able to reach, but don't be too easy on yourself, either. You may be surprised by how much you *can* do.

When you finish the book, you'll see how you can keep a record of your improving health as the weeks and months go by, as shown in the section following Chapter 5.

THE LIFE MANAGEMENT SELF-EVALUATION TEST

My Nutrition

	Points
I feel I overeat:	
Usually	0
Occasionally	1
Rarely	3
I have indigestion:	
Often	0
Occasionally	1
Rarely	3
At the table, I salt my food:	
Usually	0
Occasionally	1
Rarely	3
My refined sugar and sweet food consumption is:	
Average or above	0
Less than average	1
Very low	3
My daily sugar substitute servings are:	
Three or more	0
One or two	1
None	3

	Points
My daily alcohol consumption is:	
Three or more drinks	0
Two	1
One	2
None	3
My total weekly egg consumption in all food is:	
Ten or more	0
Eight or nine	1
Seven or less	3
My bread consumption consists of:	
White	0
Light brown/wheat	1
Whole wheat	3
My cereal consumption consists of:	
Boxed cereals, presweetened	0
Vitamin enriched (with extra roughage)	1
Whole grain	3
My daily soft drink (8 oz.) consumption is:	
Three or more	0
One or two	1
None	3
My daily tea consumption is:	
Five or more cups	0
Two to four cups	1
Two cups or less (or herbal tea)	3
My daily coffee consumption is:	
Four or more cups	0
Two or three cups	1
Decaffeinated	2
One cup or less	3

	Points
I use:	
Butter	0
Soft or liquid margarine (or none)	3
My daily roughage intake consists of:	
Normal diet	0
Extra salad and raw vegetables	1
Extra source of fiber once or twice a day	3
Meat in my diet consists mainly of:	
Fatty meats (untrimmed marbled beef, bacon, luncheon meats)	0
Meats (lean beef and pork, veal; chicken, turkey, and fish cooked with skin)	1
Lean meats (fish, chicken, turkey cooked without skin)	3
No meat at all	3
The dairy products in my diet are mostly:	
Whole milk/cream products (include most cheeses) or imitation dairy products or coconut oil	0
Low-fat dairy products	1
Skim milk or no dairy products, low-fat cheeses, low-fat yogurt	3

My nutrition score is _____

My Exercise, Occupation, Recreation, and General Fitness

Activities

	Points
My exercise program consists of:	
Little or no exercise	0
Walking program three or more days per week	1
Easy to moderate exercise three or more days per week	2
Fairly vigorous exercise in exercise attire three or more days per week	5
Heavy exercise in exercise attire three or four days per week	8
Heavy exercise in exercise attire five to seven days per week	10
My occupational activities consist of:	
Mostly mental activity with little or no manual labor	0
Combination of mental and manual labor	2
Mostly manual labor (I perspire from my work)	4
My recreational activities and hobbies consist of:	
Gardening, doubles tennis, sailing, reading, and other sedentary activities	0
Singles tennis, hiking, light bicycling and other moderately fatiguing activities	2
Prolonged and fatiguing physical activities	4

Activities score _____

Weight

The average person in good physical condition reaches a desirable weight between the ages of 18 and 23. Comparing your weight then and now, you are presently:

10	9	7	5	2	0	-2	-4	-6	-8	-10
At or below that weight	1–3 lbs. over	4–6 over	7–10 over	11–15 over	16–20 over	21–30 over	31–40 over	41–50 over	51–75 over	76 or more over

If you have always been overweight, circle how many pounds overweight you now are.

Weight score _____

Systolic blood pressure

	-5	-3	-2	-1	1	4	6	7	8	9	10
Male	180	160	150	140	135	130	125	121	118	115	110
Female, premenopause	177	157	147	137	132	127	122	119	116	113	108
Female, postmenopause	184	164	154	144	139	134	129	125	122	118	113

If not known, check here _____ and circle 4.   Systolic score _____

Diastolic blood pressure

	-5	-3	-2	-1	1	4	6	7	8	9	10
Male	99	96	93	90	88	84	80	75	70	68	65
Female, premenopause	99	95	90	88	86	83	78	73	68	66	63
Female, postmenopause	99	97	95	92	88	86	82	76	73	68	65

If not known, check here _____ and circle 4.   Diastolic score _____

My total fitness score is _____

My Personality and How I Handle Stress

	Points
I am anxious/nervous:	
Often	0
Occasionally	1
Seldom	3
I would describe myself as:	
Highly competitive	0
Moderately competitive	1
Not competitive	3
When confronted with a situation that bothers or angers me:	
I keep it to myself	0
I may or may not say something	1
I always say something about it	3
Criticism or scolding bothers me:	
Greatly	0
Moderately	1
Hardly at all	3
In my work, success is:	
Very important	0
Moderately important	1
Not important	3
I go out of my way to avoid unpleasant acquaintances:	
Often	0
Occasionally	1
Rarely	3
I have spells of the blues:	
Often	0
Occasionally	1
Rarely	3

	Points
I have disturbed sleep:	
Often	0
Occasionally	1
Rarely	3
People disappoint me:	
Often	0
Occasionally	1
Rarely	3
I am depressed:	
Often	0
Occasionally	1
Rarely	3
In my own work, I am confronted with making important decisions:	
Often	0
Occasionally	1
Seldom	3
"Our country is going to the dogs" is a statement with which I:	
Agree greatly	0
Agree moderately	1
Agree hardly at all	3
I am sexually frustrated:	
Often	0
Occasionally	1
Rarely	3
I am secretive:	
Greatly	0
Moderately	1
Hardly at all	3

My personality/stress score is _____

My Lifestyle

Basic information about myself

	Points
I have worked in a smoky office for 16 or more years	− 3
I have worked in a smoky office for 10-15 years	− 2
I have worked in a smoky office for 1-9 years	− 1
I have lived in a smoggy area such as Los Angeles for 10 or more years	− 2
I have lived in a smoggy area such as Los Angeles for 1-9 years	− 1
I have had emphysema (breathing obstruction) for 10 years or more	− 3
I have had emphysema for 1-9 years	− 1
I have had a heart attack or heart disease	− 10
I have not had a heart attack or heart disease, but have had heart or chest pain (angina)	− 5
I have or have had diabetes	− 5
I have or have had kidney disorders	− 3
I have or have had thyroid conditions	− 3
I have or have had gout	− 3
I have or have had leg cramps or claudication	− 2

Basic information score _____

Smoking and Pulmonary Status

-15	-10	-8	-5
Over 30 cigarettes per day (or inhale pipe/cigar)	21–30 cigarettes per day	10–20 cigarettes per day	1–9 cigarettes per day
-3 Over 2 cigarettes per day (or pipe/cigar, but not inhale)	**1** 20 or more cigarettes per day (or inhaled pipe/cigar), but quit less than 5 years ago		**2** 19 or less cigarettes per day, but quit less than 5 years ago
3 20 or more cigarettes per day, but quit 5–10 years ago	**5** 19 or less cigarettes per day, but quit 5–10 years ago	**6** 20 or more cigarettes per day, but quit over 10 years ago	**7** Never smoked, but lived with tobacco smoker for more than 10 years
8 Never smoked, but lived with a smoker less than 10 years		**10** 5–19 cigarettes per day, but quit over 10 years ago	**10** Never smoked or lived with a smoker

Smoking/pulmonary status score _____

Age

Male

3	0	1	2	3	4	5
72 or over	71–68	67–64	63–61	60–57	56–54	53–49

6	7	8	9	10
48–44	43–40	39–35	34–21	20 or under

Male age score _____

Female

3	2	1	0	2	4
79 or over	78–75	74–70	69–66	65–60	59–54

6	7	8	9	10
53–46	45–38	37–30	29–21	20 or under

Female age score _____

Gender

0	1	2	7	8	9	10
Male, stocky, bald	Male, stocky	Male	Female 55 or over	Female 54–50	Female 49–36	Female 35 or under

Gender score _____

Family history

I have the following number of relatives (parents and grandparents) who had heart disease, stroke, or circulatory disorder which occurred between the indicated ages:

0	1	2	3	5	10
1 or more under age 50	2 or more between 50–60 years	1 between 50–60 years	2 over 60 years	1 over 60 years	None

Family history score _____

My total lifestyle score is _____

My total score (nutrition, fitness, personality/stress, and lifestyle) is _____

How Does Your Wellness Add Up?

Extremely dangerous health risk . . . . 50 & below
Dangerous health risk 51–60
Poor health risk 61–70
Unsatisfactory health risk 71–80
Satisfactory health risk 81–90
Very good, low health risk 91–100
Excellent, very low health risk 101–120
Exceptionally low health risk . . . . Over 120

The score you achieve on this test is not a guarantee that you are absolutely a "high" or "low" health risk, since such scores are a result of statistical averages regarding various health risk factors. Your score will, however, give you a good idea of how you compare to others and where you need to concentrate your efforts at improving your health and fitness lifestyle.

This test is adapted from a risk analysis developed by Howard F. Hunt, Ph.D., and James R. White, Ph.D., of the University of California, San Diego.

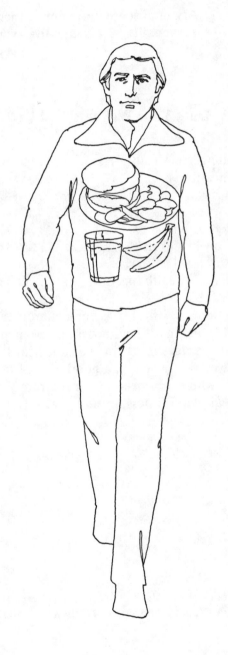

2

Nutrition

One of the greatest paradoxes in the advances of the past century is that while the average life expectancy is significantly longer than it was 100 years ago, many of the foods that we eat to sustain life have declined in quality.

It's axiomatic that we are what we eat. Every muscle, nerve, bone, and tissue of your body is made up from the foods you eat and the fluids you drink. A century ago these foods came primarily from natural sources, and they were eaten mostly in an unrefined state. Other than salt and natural spices, preservatives were largely unknown.

A large proportion of the foods we eat today have been processed. They are frozen, canned, often high in sugar and added nonnutritional substances, or heavily salted. Indeed, the great reliance on sugar and fats in the diet is one of the causes of obesity and possibly other chronic diseases. Because the food we eat affects the way we look and feel, it is important that we take a serious look at our eating habits.

The purpose of this chapter is to give you an easy, painless way to return to eating more natural, basic, and unrefined foods. With this gradual transition toward healthful eating, you will have taken a giant step toward improving your health, energy, well-being, and—very probabiy—your longevity.

OUR CHANGING DIET

The average diet has changed dramatically over the past 100 years. The proportion of meat and fat consumed has increased, while the proportion of carbohydrate intake has decreased. And what carbohydrates we do consume come from a much higher percentage of sugar and other refined sources than in the past.

This trend has resulted in a decreased intake of starch and fiber, as well as of several important vitamins and minerals. Consumption of refined sugars, fats, and alcohol has now increased to the point where about 30–40% of the average daily intake of calories comes from these empty-calorie sources—generally hidden within normal processed foods.

It is difficult to isolate the health effect of one dietary change from others, because all nutritional elements and their effects are interrelated. Therefore, it's probable that any ill health linked to dietary abuse results from a change in more than one part of your diet. As an example, an increase in sugar and fat consumption along with a decrease in fiber intake can lead to an increase in obesity. The increase in adult-onset diabetes during this century could be in part the result of increased obesity, but also might be due partly to the decreased intake of the fiber and chromium found in whole grains. Population studies show that cancers of the bowel and rectum are as closely related to low-fiber intake as to high-fat diets. High blood pressure can be provoked by increased ingestion of salted convenience foods along with a decrease in potassium-rich fruits, vegetables, grains, and legumes. Nevertheless there are many things each of us can do to improve our diet, to put it in a healthy state and keep it there.

ARE YOU EATING RIGHT?

Before considering specifics on how you can gradually and painlessly change your diet to improve your health, it would be valuable for you to determine exactly how you are eating now. Then you can set about progressively changing your dietary habits.

Before you read on, write down on the Diet History form (Table 1, pages 20–21) *everything* that you ate or drank yesterday. If you have trouble remembering, start with today's diet (but be sure to eat your normal diet).

Start your Diet History with the first thing you ate or drank in the morning. Then move through the day, ending with the last thing you consumed before going to sleep. Write down only the foods you actually ate, not how much was put on your plate.

Use standard volume measurements—cups, tablespoons, etc.— to record the amount of each food or beverage consumed. For pieces of food that cannot easily be measured with a cup or spoon, write down the approximate size (see the Sample Diet History on pages 22–23). To estimate the weight of the meat you ate, compare your portion to the palm of your hand. A piece of any kind of meat the size of a large palm would weigh about five ounces. If it's the size of a small palm, it would weigh about three ounces.

Be sure to record every ingredient contained in a mixed food. For example, if you ate a cheeseburger yesterday, list the bun, hamburger patty, cheese, lettuce, and dressing separately. Also remember to write down all the little things added to the foods you ate. These can include butter, margarine, oil, jelly, sugar, gravy, salad dressing, and other condiments and sauces. Be sure to list the snacks and drinks consumed with and between meals.

Table 2, Sample Diet History, shows how you might fill out your own form (see pages 22–23). At this point, of course, we have discussed only the left side of the form. Later you will learn how to calculate the numbers at the right side and bottom of the Diet History. By looking at the form right now you might already

TABLE 1: Diet History

Name _____   Age _____

Time	Place	Amount	Description of Foods Eaten	Number of Servings Consumed								
				Breads/Cereals {Refined	Breads/Cereals {Whole	Leafy Green Vegetables	Vitamin C-Rich Fruits & Vegetables	Other Fruits & Vegetables	Protein-Rich Foods {Animal	Protein-Rich Foods {Vegetable	Milk Products	Fats/Oils

		Total	Servings Needed	Difference

Tsp. of sugar eaten |
Tsp. "hidden" fat eaten |
No. of salty foods eaten |

TABLE 2: Sample Diet History

Name _____ John Doe _____   Age __ 44 __

Time	Place	Amount	Description of Foods Eaten	Breads/Cereals Refined	Breads/Cereals Whole	Leafy Green Vegetables	Vitamin C-Rich Fruits & Vegetables	Other Fruits & Vegetables	Protein-Rich Foods Animal	Protein-Rich Foods Vegetable	Milk Products	Fats/Oils
7:15	home	1 cup	coffee									
		2 tbs.	coffee cream									1
		2 tsp.	sugar									
		2	fried eggs						1			
		2 slices	white toast	2								
		1 tbs.	margarine									3
		1 tbs.	strawberry jam									
		2 links	sausage						½			
8:30	office	1 cup	coffee									
		1 tbs.	nondairy creamer									½
		2 tsp.	sugar									
10:00	office	1	glazed donut									
		1 cup	coffee									
		1 tbs.	nondairy creamer									½
		2 tsp.	sugar									
12:30	deli	1	kaiser roll	2				1 ½				
		1 oz.	ham									

Number of Servings Consumed

		2 oz.	American cheese								1¼	
		1 tbs.	mayonnaise									3
		¼ cup	shredded iceberg lettuce					¼				
		2 slices	onion					¼				
		¼ cup	shredded cabbage			¼						
		1 tbs.	cole slaw dressing									2
		1 cup	french fried potatoes					2				
		2 tbs.	catsup									
		12 oz.	cola									
3:30	office	1	chocolate candy bar									
5:00	home	4 oz.	bourbon (with water)									
		½ cup	peanuts							1		
7:00	home	1 cup	white rice	2								
		2 tsp.	margarine									2
		8 oz.	broiled steak						4			
		½ cup	canned green peas					1				
		½ cup	iceberg lettuce					1				
		½ med.	tomato				¼					
		½ cup	blue cheese dressing									8
9:00	home	1½ cups	ice cream								1	
		4 med.	chocolate chip cookies									
10:00	home	10 oz.	whole milk								1¼	
Tsp. of sugar eaten		37	Total	6	0	¼	¼	4½	7	1	3½	20
Tsp. "hidden" fat eaten		41	Servings Needed	2	2	1	2	3	1	1	2	4
No. of salty foods eaten		5	Difference	+4	−2	−¾	−1¾	+1½	+6	0	+1½	+16

be able to see graphically what foods you are eating and where you can change your diet for the better.

Let's now begin to explore realistically whether you should modify your diet to improve your health and fitness.

EAT A VARIETY OF FOODS

Most people have a bad habit of eating the same 10-12 foods over and over again. This is very unhealthy, since no single food item supplies all the essential nutrients in the amounts needed for optimal health. Even combinations of 10-12 foods are likely to be deficient in several vital nutrients. Therefore, it is necessary to eat a fairly wide variety of foods to assure an adequate diet. The greater the variety of foods you eat, the less likely it is that you will develop either a deficiency or an excess of any single nutrient.

One way to obtain variety in your eating, and with it a well-balanced diet, is to select foods each day from seven main groups. In Table 3, Daily Food Guide, foods are divided into several groups by composition and nutritional value (see opposite page). Meals chosen from the minimum servings in this guide will supply at least 80 percent of the recommended amount for all nutrients with Recommended Dietary Allowances (RDAs) assigned. The remainder will come from other foods not specifically listed and from additional servings from the Daily Food Guide.

Some of the most difficult nutrients to obtain in adequate amounts are vitamin B-6, folic acid, magnesium, and zinc. Including some vegetable protein foods and whole grains in your daily diet will assure you an adequate supply of these nutrients. Also, the protein food servings recommended in the Daily Food Guide are often higher than the amount actually needed to supply enough protein in order to ensure an adequate intake of vitamin B-6, iron, and zinc.

Let's assume, for purposes of illustration, that your Diet History will look the same as the Sample Diet History. Compare the Sample Diet History with the Daily Food Guide to see whether you got the minimum number of servings of each food group sug-

TABLE 3: Daily Food Guide

Food Group	Good Sources of These Nutrients	One Serving Equals	Recommended Minimum Servings			
			Child (2-10 yrs.)	Teen (11-18 yrs.)	Adult (19+ yrs.)	Pregnant/ Breast-feeding
BREADS AND CEREALS Whole-grain and enriched breads, cereals, rolls, tortillas, noodles, spaghetti, macaroni, pancakes, waffles, muffins; oatmeal, rice, barley, bulgur or cracked wheat.	All provide carbohydrates and some protein. (Protein quality improved when eaten together with Protein-Rich Foods or Milk Products listed below.) All provide thiamin, niacin, riboflavin and iron. Whole grains provide additional vitamin B-6, folic acid, vitamin E, magnesium, zinc and fiber.	1 slice of bread; 1 dinner roll; ½ bun or English muffin; 1 tortilla; ¾ cup of dry cereal; ½ cup of cooked cereal, rice or noodles; 1 tbs. of wheat germ; 1 5″ pancake or waffle; 1 muffin.	4	5	4	5
				(Try to have 2-3 servings from whole-grain products.)		
LEAFY GREEN VEGETABLES Romaine, red leaf lettuce; chard, collards, dandelion, kale, spinach, turnip, and other greens; broccoli, brussels sprouts, cabbage; asparagus; parsley, watercress, scallions (green onions), fresh mint.	Excellent sources of folic acid, vitamins A and B-6, riboflavin and magnesium. Also supply good amounts of iron, potassium, and fiber.	1 cup raw; ¾ cup cooked.	½-1	1	1	1-2

VITAMIN C-RICH FRUITS AND VEGETABLES Citrus, tomatoes, berries, melons (cantaloupe, mango, papaya), peppers, cabbage, cauliflower, broccoli, brussels sprouts.	Excellent sources of vitamin C and potassium. Also supply folic acid, vitamin A and fiber.	1 orange; ½ grapefruit or melon; 2 lemons; 2 tomatoes; ½ cup of sliced fruit or vegetable; ½ cup of orange or grapefruit juice; 1½ cups of tomato juice.	1	2	2	2
OTHER FRUITS AND VEGETABLES Corn, carrots, green beans, iceberg (head) lettuce, peas, potatoes, apples, bananas, peaches, pears; raisins and other dried fruits; and all other fruits and vegetables not on the preceding two lists.	Provide carbohydrates, fiber and potassium, as well as smaller amounts of other essential vitamins and minerals. If deep orange and/or yellow, also excellent sources of vitamin A. Raisins are good source of iron.	1 medium piece of fruit or vegetable; ½ cup of sliced raw or cooked fruit or vegetable; 2 tbs. of dried fruits	2	3	3	3
PROTEIN-RICH FOODS Animal: meat, poultry, seafood, eggs, hot dogs, luncheon meats, sausage. Vegetable: dried beans, lentils, split peas, peanuts, peanut butter, nuts.	All are excellent sources of protein, iron, vitamin B-6, zinc. All animal protein supplies vitamin B-12. Seafood supplies iodine and selenium. Vegetable protein supplies folic acid, vitamin E and magnesium.	2 oz. cooked lean meat, poultry, seafood; 2 eggs; 2 hot dogs; 3 slices luncheon meat; 4 links sausage; 3 fish sticks; 1 cup cooked beans; ½ cup peanuts or nuts; 4 tbs. of peanut butter.	1-2	3-4	2	4

(Try to have 1-2 servings from vegetable foods high in protein).

MILK PRODUCTS

Milk; kefir, yogurt; cheese, custard, ice cream, milk-based puddings; tofu (soybean curd).

All are excellent sources of protein and calcium. In addition, milk products are good sources of vitamins A, B-12 and riboflavin. Fortified fluid milk contains 100 IU of vitamin D per cup. Cheese is a good source of zinc.

1 cup of milk, kefir, yogurt; 1½ slices of pre-sliced American cheese, 1½ oz. or ⅓ cup grated brick-type cheese (like Cheddar or Jack); 5 tbs. of Parmesan; 1¼ cups of Cottage cheese; 1 cup of custard; 1½ cups of ice cream; 1 cup of pudding; 1 cup of tofu (contains no vitamin B-12 or D).

2   3   2   4

FATS AND OILS

Butter, margarine, vegetable oil, mayonnaise, salad dressing; cream; seeds; avocadoes, olives; bacon.

Provide energy because of the fats they contain. The polyunsaturated vegetable oils and seeds are good sources of the essential fatty acids and moderate to good sources of vitamin E.

1 tsp. of butter, margarine, oil, mayonnaise; ½ tbs. of salad dressing; 2 tbs. of sour cream or coffee cream; 1 tbs. of whipping cream; 2 tsp. of sesame or sunflower seeds; 1/8 avocado; 5 small olives; 1 slice of bacon.

3   4   4   5

Source: Modified from the chapter "Nutritional Prevention" by Vicky Newman in *Practice of Preventative Health Care* by Larry Schiederman (Menlo Park, Cal.: Addison-Wesley Publishing Co., 1981).

gested for you. For example, adults need a minimum of four servings daily from the breads and cereals (refined and whole) group. If you ate two slices of white toast (which equals two servings), one kaiser roll (which equals two servings), and one cup of cooked rice (which also equals two servings), you consumed a total of six servings from the breads and cereals group, or two more than the recommended minimum number of servings for adults. As another example, adults need a minimum of two servings from the combined animal and vegetable protein-rich foods group. If you ate two fried eggs (which equals one serving of protein-rich food), two sausage links (which equals half of a serving), a half-cup of peanuts (which equals one serving), and an eight-ounce broiled steak (which equals four servings), you ate a total of eight servings of protein-rich foods from both animal and vegetable sources. This is substantially more than the recommended minimum of two servings for adults.

Notice that the servings recommended are the minimal amounts required by an average-sized person. If you consume this minimum number of servings and you can afford taking in extra calories, go ahead and eat either larger portions of these foods or foods that are not listed. For optimum health, however, it would be best if most of the foods you eat come from the Daily Food Guide.

CALORIES AND MAINTENANCE—YOUR IDEAL WEIGHT

We eat approximately as many calories today as we did at the beginning of the century, but we use fewer calories because we are much less active. A larger proportion of the calories we consume comes from refined sugars, starches, and fats, which aggravate obesity problems. These calories are more efficiently absorbed by the body than are calories from unrefined fibrous foods like whole grains, vegetables, fruits, and legumes (dried peas, beans, and lentils).

Eating and absorbing more calories than we burn causes the body to store energy in the form of fat. Being obese not only may make us feel unattractive but also makes regular work and recreation harder. Obesity is a major risk factor in the development of such chronic diseases as diabetes, high blood pressure, heart disease, and certain forms of cancer. Thus, the maintenance of an ideal body weight is of vital importance. Most individuals should maintain throughout life the weight they had reached at age 18, when maximum skeletal growth is normally achieved.

If it's necessary to lose fat weight, a gradual and steady loss of one or two pounds per week is recommended. Not only is a weight loss at this rate more likely to be maintained for a long period of time, but you are also more likely to follow a nutritionally balanced diet on a more moderate reducing regimen. Long-term success in losing weight depends on your gradually acquiring new and better dietary and exercise habits. Exercise is discussed at length in the following chapter, so suffice it to point out here that exercise burns off calories. You should try to integrate your dietary patterns with the type of regular exercise you get. If you want to lose weight, that means you should begin a twofold program that strengthens your muscles through proper exercise and reduces body weight through foods lower in calories and higher in good nutritional content. This is undoubtedly why crash diets are rarely successful in the long run.

It's best to avoid diets containing fewer than 1,200 calories per day; diets of 800 calories or fewer per day may actually be hazardous to your health.

Excessive weight loss—to 85 percent or less of one's ideal weight—may result in menstrual irregularities, infertility, hair loss, skin changes, cold intolerance, and severe constipation. Besides trying to lose fat too quickly, many individuals—particularly women—are trying to become too thin.

It's important not to go to opposite extremes in losing weight. Make sure you know what *your* ideal body weight is. Crash diets are rough on your body, and virtually no one who loses weight on a crash diet is able to keep it off. Instead of crash dieting, aim for a slow, gradual, and progressive modification of your eating patterns.

While reading this chapter you are learning what not to eat and which foods you can substitute for those that do little or nothing to promote good health. But don't make such substitutions overnight. Progress slowly and comfortably, changing a food here and there and even briefly enjoying a small portion every week or two of some food you shouldn't be eating. In this way you'll be able to make significant and long-lasting changes in your diet without discomfort.

Approximating Your Ideal Body Weight

Medium Frame
Males: Start with 106 pounds for the first five feet and add six pounds for each inch thereafter. (For example, if you are a 5'10" male of medium frame, your ideal body weight is 166 pounds.)

Females: Start with 100 pounds for the first five feet and add five pounds for each inch thereafter. (For example, if you are a 5'4" female of medium frame, your ideal body weight is 120 pounds.)

Small Frame
If you have a small frame or are small-boned, subtract 10 percent from the total obtained above.

Large Frame
If you have a large frame or are large-boned, add 10 percent to your total.

Tips for the Calorie-Conscious

Simply increasing your intake of fiber-rich fruits, vegetables, whole grains, and legumes—while decreasing your intake of fatty meat, sugar, fat, and alcohol—will help immensely in weight control. Additional practical ideas for decreasing your sugar and fat intake will be presented later in this chapter.

Limiting your daily intake to the suggested servings on the Daily Food Guide (Table 3) and following the suggestions below can help you cut calories to lose weight and keep it off.

Breads and Cereals

- Emphasize whole-grain breads and cereals (whole wheat bread and oatmeal, for example).
- Avoid sweetened breads and cereals.
- Avoid those made with added fat (muffins, pancakes, waffles).
- You might want to cut down to three servings daily.

Leafy Green Vegetables

- Eat these in unlimited quantities.
- Fill up on them when you're hungry.
- Occasionally make a meal that consists of a large green salad.

Vitamin C-Rich Fruits and Vegetables

- Choose fruits rather than juices. (You'll feel full on fewer calories.)
- Eat these vegetables in unlimited quantities.

Other Fruits and Vegetables

- Eat fried vegetables sparingly.
- Avoid vegetables with added sauces.
- Count each banana as two servings.

Protein-Rich Foods

- Choose only the leanest cuts of meat and trim away any visible fat before eating.
- Bake, broil, grill, or boil; don't fry.
- Avoid high-fat processed meats (hot dogs, luncheon meats, sausages, and so on).
- Decrease use of peanuts and other nuts, peanut butter.

Milk Products

- Cut down on high-fat milk; emphasize low-fat or skim.
- Use cheeses made from part skim milk.
- Reduce intake of sweetened milk products (e.g., fruited yogurt, custard, ice cream, pudding).

Fats and Oils

- Carefully measure all of these. (The calories are very concentrated.)
- You might want to cut down to two servings daily of foods high in fats and oils.

Diet and Exercise

Diet and exercise make a good one-two punch when fighting the battle of the bulge. A reduction of caloric content in the diet, particularly when coupled with regular sessions of aerobic exercise, can be very effective in helping you to achieve and maintain ideal body weight. In a brisk aerobic activity like dancing, swimming, jogging, or cycling, you will burn 50–100 calories in only 10 minutes.

Many individuals make the mistake of thinking that they can continue to eat high-calorie foods as long as they're careful to exercise every day. This is a fallacy, however, because it's much easier to reduce body fat levels dietetically than through exercise. Depending on how heavy a person is, he or she can burn 100–120 calories by running 1 mile. But that same person can avoid consuming those 100–120 calories in the first place merely by refusing to eat a pat of butter on a potato or to put a tablespoon of oil on a salad.

You would have to run nearly 4 miles to burn off the calories in a cup of ice cream, 1 mile for a single plain donut, more than 3 miles for a slice of apple pie, and a little under 20 miles to burn off the calories in an average porterhouse steak. Thus, while you should resolve to exercise regularly for the sake of better health and muscle tone, keep in mind that you would make even more progress if you combined a sound, moderate diet with a sound, moderate exercise program.

An added benefit of combining diet with exercise to lose weight is that exercise is best done on lower calorie foods, particularly on carbohydrates. Instead of devouring a huge steak as a pregame meal, as athletes did in the past, today's athletes munch on fruit and other carbohydrate food that will supply them with quick energy during the game. Fruits have readily available carbohydrates, but overall are quite low in calories. When you exercise consistently, your body instinctively craves low calorie natural carbohydrates, such as fruits, to satisfy its energy needs.

If you continue exercising for a minimum of 30 minutes, you get the added benefit of elevating your basal metabolic rate (BMR) for several additional hours. So you not only burn calories while exercising; you also use more than the usual number of calories for several hours after ceasing to exercise.

DEVELOP GOOD EATING HABITS

Eat More Unrefined Carbohydrates

As mentioned earlier in this chapter, the consumption of all types of carbohydrates has declined during the past century. But perhaps as important is the fact that the type of carbohydrates we consume has shifted from primarily starches—potatoes, legumes, and grains—to primarily sugars (sweets and soft drinks). Also, unrefined carbohydrates—whole grains, fresh whole potatoes, salads, fruits, and vegetables—have increasingly been replaced by their refined counterparts. Such products as white flour, potato chips, and juice "drinks" (which contain loads of sugar and less than 10 percent natural juice) are far inferior to their natural counterparts.

Perhaps one of the reasons carbohydrate consumption has decreased is that people think of carbohydrates as being fattening. Actually, ounce for ounce they contain less than half the calories that fat contains: one gram of fat equals nine calories when metabolized for energy in the human body; one gram of carbohydrate yields only four calories. Replacing fats, fried foods, and fatty meats in your diet with unrefined fruits, vegetables, grains, and legumes will help you control your weight by preventing over-consumption of calories. For example, steak is often fatty and therefore contains a great number of calories in relation to its volume. A highly marbled 12-ounce steak can have the same number of calories as nine medium-size baked potatoes. And, obviously, nine potatoes are a lot bulkier than the steak.

Unrefined carbohydrates also contain significant amounts of plant fiber, which has recently been suggested as playing a role in the prevention of cancer of the colon and certain other chronic diseases. When plant fiber is removed from a grain, vegetable, or fruit to make white flour, white sugar, or juices, calories are concentrated. Because concentrated calories can be consumed quickly, there is a counterproductive tendency to ingest many more calories before a sense of fullness is noticed. This would be less likely if foods were eaten in their natural forms. As an example, a 12-ounce glass of apple juice contains about the same number of calories as three apples. Wouldn't you feel full or grow tired of chewing before you consumed three apples? Yet you can gulp down a glass of apple juice so quickly that it probably wouldn't even begin to make you feel full.

A piece of apple pie—because of sugar and other ingredients—contains roughly the same number of calories as seven apples, but think of how fast you can eat that piece of pie compared to chomping down seven apples!

Plant fiber also appears to protect people from certain discomforts and diseases. Populations that eat diets plentiful in fiber-rich foods seem to experience less constipation, hemorrhoids, and diverticulosis (intestinal pouches that can become inflamed).

Fiber-rich foods contain a number of different kinds of fibers. Some types are more effective in decreasing fat absorption and lowering cholesterol levels than others. Cholesterol is a fat-like substance found in animal products and also produced in our own bodies. Some cholesterol is necessary for normal body functioning, but excessive amounts in the blood are risk factors for heart disease. As an example, purified cellulose (added to certain refined breads) and bran are both relatively ineffective in lowering the cholesterol level of your blood. However, oatmeal and pectin—as well as gums and lignin—have a cholesterol-lowering effect. Pectin is plentiful in such fruits as apples and citrus. Gums and lignin are found in grains, legumes, and vegetables. Several studies have particularly noted the cholesterol-lowering properties of legumes (dried peas, beans, and lentils).

Studies of various populations suggest that a diet high in fiber may provide protection from cancer of the colon (large intestine) and rectum. Fiber is thought to exert its apparent effect on the carcinogenic process in several ways. It increases fecal bulk and decreases transit time. This in turn is said to reduce the concentration of cancer-causing substances in the intestine and decreases the time that the intestinal lining is exposed to these substances. For more information on the dietary fiber content of various fibrous foods, see Table 4 (pages 36–37).

In addition to concentrating calories and removing fiber, the refining and processing of grains, fruits, and vegetables results in the loss of important vitamins and minerals. For instance, much of the vitamin B-6, folic acid, pantothenic acid, magnesium, and zinc is removed when grains are milled. Thiamin, niacin, riboflavin, and iron are also removed, but these are added back into many enriched products such as cereals and breads.

Take a look at your Diet History again. Did you eat the recommended minimum number of servings from the leafy green, vitamin C-rich, and other fruit and vegetable groups? Did you eat enough breads, whole-grain foods, and cereals? How about legumes in the protein-rich group?

TABLE 4: Dietary Fiber Content of Selected Foods

Food	Serving Size	Fiber/Serving (grams)
Breads/Crackers		
Crispbread, rye	2 crackers	1.48
White bread	1 slice	0.63
Whole wheat bread	1 slice	1.96
Breakfast Cereals		
Bran cereals	¾ cup	11.20
Cornflakes	¾ cup	2.09
Oatmeal, cooked	1 cup	3.22
Shredded wheat	1 biscuit	2.70
Flours		
White	½ cup	1.89
Whole wheat	½ cup	6.28
Bran	1/8 cup or 2 tablespoons	3.30
Fruits		
Apple (with skin)	1 medium	2.41
Banana	1 6-inch	1.75
Cherries	25 small or 15 large	1.24
Orange	1 medium	2.85
Peach (with skin)	1 medium	2.28
Pear (with skin)	1 medium	2.07
Plums (with skin)	2 medium	1.52
Strawberries (raw)	10 large	2.12
Legumes		
Beans (baked) canned	½ cup	9.27
Beans (green) boiled	½ cup	1.67
Peas (frozen) raw	½ cup	5.66
Peas (canned)	½ cup	5.26
Nuts		
Peanuts	¼ cup	3.36

Food	Serving Size	Fiber/Serving (grams)
Vegetables (Leafy)		
Broccoli tops (boiled)	½ cup	2.99
Brussels sprouts	½ cup	2.00
Cabbage	½ cup	2.07
Cauliflower	½ cup	1.13
Lettuce (raw)	½ cup	0.84
Onions (raw)	1 2¼-inch diameter	2.10
Vegetables (Root)		
Carrots (young) boiled	½ cup	2.78
Corn (canned)	½ cup	4.72
Corn (cooked)	1 ear	4.74
Parsnips (raw)	½ large	4.90
Peppers (cooked)	½ cup	0.63
Potato (canned)	½ cup	3.13
Potato (raw)	1 2¼-inch diameter	3.51
Tomatoes (canned)	½ cup	1.02
Tomatoes (fresh)	1 small	1.40
Turnips (raw)	⅔ cup	1.89

Source: Derived from *Handbook of Clinical Dietetics*, American Dietetic Association (New Haven, Conn.: Yale University Press, 1981).

You'll be surprised at how good fresh bread, legumes, vegetables, and unsweetened fruit can taste! Eat slowly. Savor the taste and texture of these delicious foods!

Tips on Increasing Intake of Unrefined Carbohydrates

- Increase your intake of legumes (dried peas, beans, lentils), potatoes, and other vegetables.
- Eat whole-grain breads and cereals daily.
- Be sure the labels on breads and cereals list whole wheat or grains as the first ingredient.

- Keep in mind that the term *wheat flour* on bread labels means white flour.
- If you don't like whole wheat bread, eat old-fashioned oatmeal or a whole-grain cold cereal in the morning.
- Consume whole fresh fruits instead of fruit juices or fruit drinks.
- If fresh fruit is not available, of low quality, or too expensive, try fruit frozen without added sugar. Berries are usually available this way.
- Try to eat a fruit or vegetable—preferably fresh—with each meal. It's preferable for these to come from the dark green leafy and vitamin C-rich groups (see Daily Food Guide).
- Along with the traditional carrots and celery, try wedges of cabbage, flowerets of broccoli or cauliflower, slices of turnips or rutabagas.
- Try to serve two different vegetables with dinner in addition to a starchy grain or potato and a salad.

Eat Less Sugar

According to the U.S. Department of Agriculture, the average person consumes approximately 130 pounds of all types of refined sugars and sweeteners in a year—other than those sugars eaten in certain natural fruits. That's about 36 teaspoons of sweeteners every day of the year!

Much of this sugar comes from soft drinks. For example, each 12-ounce can of soda contains about nine teaspoons of sugar. There is abundant evidence that our large intake of sugar is one of several factors that can predispose us to tooth decay and obesity.

Take a look at your Diet History. How much sugar did you consume? Check Table 5 to help you approximate your sugar intake. Use a pen to circle any foods in your Diet History chart that appear on this list. Then add up your sugar intake. Mark the total in the space provided at the bottom of your form.

Were you anywhere near the average American intake of 36 teaspoons of sweeteners per day? If so, you'd probably feel a lot better if you tried to cut back on your sugar consumption. For some

TABLE 5: Sugar Content of Selected Foods

Food	Serving Size	Sugar/Serving (approx. tsps.)
Cake, plain	1 slice	6
Cake, iced	1 slice	10
Candy bar	1½ ounces	2
Cereal, sweetened	½ cup	1–3
Coffeecake	1 piece	4
Cookies	2 small	3
Donut, plain	1 medium	3
Donut, glazed	1 medium	6
Fruit, canned with syrup	½ cup	3
Gelatin, plain	1 cup	12
Gelatin, with fruit	1 cup	7
Honey	1 tablespoon	4
Jam or jelly	1 tablespoon	3
Ice cream	1 cup	7
Ice cream cone	1 medium	2
Pie, fruit	1 slice	7
Pie, custard cream	1 slice	4
Pudding	1 cup	4
Sherbet	1 cup	14
Soda pop	12-ounce can	9
Sugar, syrup, molasses	1 tablespoon	3

helpful suggestions on how to cut back on your sugar intake, read on.

Tips on Reducing Refined Sugar Intake

- Use less of all sweeteners, including white sugar, brown sugar, raw sugar, honey, fructose, and syrups.
- Avoid adding sugar to coffee and tea.
- Try decreasing the amount of sweetener in your favorite recipes by one-third to one-half.

- Eat less of foods containing sweeteners, such as candy, soft drinks, ice cream, cakes, cookies, and pies.
    > At snack time, munch on fruit and raw vegetables, whole grains, and/or low-fat dairy products instead.
    > After meals, substitute fruit and/or milk desserts.
    > If you do use canned fruits, be sure to choose those that are canned in their own juice or in light syrup rather than heavy syrup.
    > Drink water instead of sweetened beverages during and between meals.
    > Try replacing soda pop with a mixture of half soda water and half fruit juice.
- Read food labels for clues on sugar content. If the words *sucrose, glucose, dextrose, fructose, corn syrup/sweeteners, maltose,* or *lactose* appear first, then there is a large amount of sugar in the product. Try to reduce intake of foods that list one of these sweeteners as a main ingredient.

Eat More Vegetable Foods

During this century the total protein food intake of the average person has remained approximately the same. However, the source of this protein food intake has changed. Early in the century, half of the protein food came from grains, legumes, potatoes, and other vegetable sources. The other half came from animal products.

Gradually the average diet has moved far more toward consumption of animal products. This trend has contributed to both an increase in fat and a decrease in carbohydrate and fiber in the average diet.

The average person also eats about twice the amount of proteins daily that his or her body requires for building and repairing tissues. The extra protein is either burned as energy or changed into fat and stored within the body. So cutting down on animal protein portions can help to save calories and fat, both in and on the body. Buying less meat can also save money in the family food budget.

Again, take a look at your Diet History. Did you eat the recommended minimum number of servings of protein-rich foods or many more? Did you eat any vegetable protein foods, such as legumes, nuts, or seeds?

If you're eating more animal protein foods than you expected, try cutting down the portions of these foods. If you are still hungry, fill up on more potatoes, grains, and vegetables.

Try eating some vegetarian meals each week. A combination of grains (like rice, wheat, or corn) and legumes or the addition of milk or eggs to an otherwise totally vegetable or grain meal will result in a high-quality protein combination equivalent to animal protein. Some vegetarian meals you might try are listed next. For more ideas and recipes, see the *Eater's Guide* and *Laurel's Kitchen,* two books listed in the Recommended Reading list at the end of this chapter.

Ideas for Vegetarian Meals

- A hearty bean or split pea soup with cornbread and a mixed vegetable salad.
- Baked beans with brown bread and an apple/carrot salad.
- Black-eyed peas with cornbread and greens (collards, kale).
- Beans with tortillas or rice and a green salad.
- Spaghetti with tomato sauce and a little cheese.
- Oatmeal with milk and a banana.
- A mixed vegetable salad with a hard-boiled egg and bread.

Eat Less Fat (Especially Less Saturated Fat)

The proportion of fat we consume has increased during this century, and most of this increased intake has been in the form of refined fats and oils, particularly margarines and salad oils. High-fat meals are also high-calorie meals, which can lead to obesity. High-fat meals also take longer to digest, which can lead to sleepiness and lethargy after eating, as well as to heartburn.

The relationship between heart disease and fat centers on the effect of different types of fats on cholesterol levels in the blood.

Saturated fats are solid at room temperature and tend to raise blood cholesterol. Such fats are found predominantly in meats and dairy products as well as in certain vegetable fats such as palm oil, coconut oil, and cocoa butter. Check for these fats on the labels of all foods that you buy.

The monounsaturated fats are liquid at room temperature but get thick when refrigerated. They neither raise nor lower blood cholesterol. Olives, peanuts, avocadoes, and most nuts (except walnuts) are high in monounsaturated fats. The polyunsaturated fats are liquid at room temperature and remain so even when refrigerated. These tend to lower blood cholesterol levels. Safflower, sunflower, and corn oils are all very high in polyunsaturated fats, while soybean oil, walnut, sesame, and cottonseed oil are less so.

Hydrogenated fats are found in margarines, shortenings, and processed foods listing hydrogenated or partially hardened vegetable oils on their ingredient lists. These fats are made by adding hydrogen to liquid oil. The more hydrogen that is added, the more saturated these oils become and, therefore, the more solid they are at room temperature. The more saturated these margarines and shortenings are, the more they tend to raise blood cholesterol levels.

When you eat margarine, pick one whose label lists liquid oil first. This shows that it contains more polyunsaturated oil than hydrogenated oil. The margarine would, therefore, have fewer of the negative characteristics associated with hydrogenation.

It's time to take another look at your Diet History form. Did you get more servings from the fats and oils group than the recommended minimum? How many extra teaspoons of fat were hidden in the foods that you ate? Count up the number of teaspoons of hidden fat that you ate yesterday. (Hidden fats are listed in Table 6.) Mark the total number in the space provided at the bottom of your Diet History form.

Tips on Reducing Fat (Especially Saturated Fat)
Did you find that you are eating more fat than you had ex-

TABLE 6: Some Foods with Hidden Fats

Food	Serving Size	Fat/Serving (approx. tsps.)
Breads/Cereals		
Biscuit	1 2-inch diameter	1
Cornbread	2x2x1-inch	1
Crackers, buttery	5	1
Danish	1 medium	3
Donut	1 medium	1½
Granola	¼ cup	1
Muffin, plain	1 2-inch diameter	1
Pancake or waffle	1 5x½-inch	1
Milk Products		
Cheese, whole milk	1 ounce	2
Cheese, part skim milk	1 ounce	1
Milk, low-fat	1 cup	1
Milk, whole	1 cup	2
Protein Foods (Animal)		
Hamburger, commercial	1 ounce	1
Hot dog	1 medium	2
Luncheon meat	1 slice	1½
Sausage	1 link	1½
Steak or chop	1 ounce	1
Protein Foods (Vegetable)		
Almonds	10 whole	1
Pecans	5 halves	1
Peanuts	2 T. or 1/8 cup	3
Peanut butter	2 T. or 1/8 cup	3
Nuts, all others not named	6 small	1
Sweets		
Cake, plain	2x3x2-inch	1½
Cake, iced	2x3x2-inch	2
Candy bar	1½ ounces	2
Cheese cake	1 slice	3
Cookie	2 2-inch diameter	1

Food	Serving Size	Fat/Serving (approx. tsps.)
Ice cream, regular	1 cup	3
Ice cream, rich	1 cup	5
Ice milk	1 cup	1
Pie	1/6 9-inch diameter	3½
Miscellaneous		
Potato chips	15	2
French fries	12 3x½x½-inch	3
Gravy (all types)	¼ cup	3
Sauce, cheese	¼ cup	2
Sauce, white	¼ cup	2

pected? If you would like to decrease your fat consumption, try to follow the tips below.

- Limit beef, pork, lamb, and whole milk cheese consumption to a combined total of 20 ounces per week. (Each ounce contains approximately one teaspoon of saturated fat.)
- When you do eat meat, select the leanest cuts and remove all visible fat before eating.
- Use poultry, fish, and legumes to replace red meat several times a week.
- Try to avoid luncheon meats, frankfurters, and sausage because they are so high in fat and salt.
- Skim the fat off broths, soups, and gravies.
- Bake, broil, grill, and boil meats. Try to avoid frying.
- Switch to nonfat or low-fat milk.
    Whole milk contains the equivalent of two teaspoons of butter per cup.
    Low-fat milk contains only about one teaspoon of butter per cup.
    Nonfat or skim milk contains no butter.
    If you prefer whole milk, you can reduce your intake of fats from other sources.

- Try to use cheeses made with part skim milk rather than those made with whole milk. Recommended cheeses include Cottage, Farmers, Ricotta, Parmesan, Mozzarella, Gruyère, Sapsago, Edam, Gouda.
- Decrease rich dishes made with butter and cream and try not to use products made with palm oil, coconut oil, and/or cocoa butter.
- Avoid food products bearing the term *hardened* or *hydrogenated* vegetable oil.
- Use only small portions of fresh butter, margarine (listing liquid oil as the first ingredient), and mayonnaise as spreads.
- Use salad dressings sparingly. (One tablespoon can contain as much as 200 calories of fat.)

Avoid Too Much Cholesterol

Most people are used to hearing that they should limit their dietary intake of cholesterol. While this plays a role in maintaining normal cholesterol levels, it is only a quarter of the dietary solution to a very complicated problem. It is important to understand that there are other food factors that affect blood cholesterol. These are: (1) excessive calories; (2) inadequate fiber; and (3) excessive fat, particularly saturated fat.

Caloric intake is a problem if it leads to excess weight gain, since obesity is associated with elevated blood cholesterol levels. Consuming fiber-rich foods helps decrease blood cholesterol levels by decreasing the absorption of cholesterol and saturated fat by the digestive system and increasing their excretion from the body. A diet rich in saturated fats tends to increase blood cholesterol levels. Recently, several studies have indicated that fresh cholesterol (as found in fresh eggs) may not raise blood cholesterol levels at all or certainly raises them much less than previously thought.

Tips on Lowering Blood Cholesterol Levels

Following the tips listed here will help you lower your blood cholesterol to the recommended level.

- Follow suggestions made elsewhere in this chapter to maintain ideal weight, increase intake of fiber-rich foods, and decrease intake of saturated fats.
- Reduce dietary cholesterol intake in two ways:
    Eat moderate amounts of animal protein foods (meat, fish, poultry, and cheese) to a combined total of six ounces daily. (Each ounce contains 25 milligrams of cholesterol.)
    Limit egg consumption to an average of one a day. Such severe restriction is unnecessary if you are a premenopausal woman or a child.

Alcohol and Coffee

Alcoholic beverages generally are high in calories and low in other nutrients. Even moderate drinkers may need to drink less if they wish to achieve ideal body weight. On the other hand, heavy drinkers may lose their appetites for foods containing essential nutrients. Vitamin and mineral deficiencies commonly occur in heavy drinkers, in part because of poor intake of food, but also because alcohol alters the absorption and use of some essential nutrients. Heavy drinking may ultimately lead to cirrhosis of the liver, neurological disorders, and a predisposition toward cancer of the throat.

Sustained or excessive alcohol consumption by pregnant women is associated with an increased risk of birth defects. Because of this risk, it's recommended that pregnant women avoid alcoholic beverages.

Moderation in caffeine consumption is advisable, chiefly because of the well-documented relationship between excessive intake and anxiety, gastritis, and heartburn.

Tips on Limiting Alcohol and Caffeine Consumption

- If you drink, limit alcoholic beverage consumption to a daily total of one ounce of absolute alcohol. This would be found in approximately two ounces of hard liquor, two five-ounce glasses of wine, or two 12-ounce cans of beer.

- If you consume caffeine drinks, limit your intake to 200 milligrams daily, which is the pharmacologically active dose. This amount would be found in approximately two five-ounce cups of coffee, four five-ounce cups of tea, or four 12-ounce cans of cola beverage.

Nutrition and High Blood Pressure: Sodium and Potassium

Sodium consumption has increased dramatically during the past century. Because sodium has a high affinity for water, it can hold 50 times its weight in water within the body's tissues. Potassium, on the other hand, helps to normalize the body's degree of water retention. Common table salt (sodium chloride), and foods to which salt has been added, is our largest source of dietary sodium.

Results of studies have shown that sodium plays an important role in the development of high blood pressure (hypertension). Approximately one out of every five adults suffers from hypertension, but less than one-half of them are aware of it. Once a disease associated with mature individuals, high blood pressure has become increasingly common among children and young adults. In addition, hypertension is a significant risk factor in heart disease. Left untreated, hypertension can lead to heart attack, stroke, or kidney failure.

While it has long been known that an excess intake of sodium can cause high blood pressure, the ability of potassium to help prevent hypertension has only recently been discovered. In the process of refining foods, we are actually increasing their sodium content and decreasing their potassium content. And this has led to the increased incidence of hypertension over the past two to three decades.

In your diet you should avoid, or at least severely curtail, your intake of sodium-rich foods (see the following section for a list of salty foods) and limit your use of table salt. At the same time you should increase your intake of potassium-rich foods, such as all fruits, fresh vegetables (particularly those prepared with no salt), legumes, and unsalted nuts and seeds.

Again, take a look at your Diet History chart. Did you eat a lot of salty foods yesterday? Check the list of salty foods that follows and circle any of those that you find on your Diet History form. Did you eat more of these foods than you realized? Mark the total number of salty foods you ate yesterday in the space provided at the bottom of your form.

Salty Foods

- Canned soups, stews, vegetables; bouillon cubes.
- Crackers with salted tops.
- Egg substitutes.
- Instant cocoa mixes.
- Pickled vegetables (olives, pickles, relishes, sauerkraut).
- Salted peanut butter.
- Salty cheeses (processed cheeses and cheese spreads; Roquefort, Camembert, Gorgonzola).
- Salty or smoked meats (bacon, bologna and other luncheon meats, chipped beef, corned beef, hot dogs, ham, meats koshered by salting, salt pork, sausage, smoked tongue).
- Salty or smoked seafood (anchovies, caviar, salt cod, herring, sardines).
- Sauces (barbecue sauce, catsup, chili sauce, steak sauce, soy sauce).
- Seasonings (celery, garlic, or onion salt; MSG; cooking wines).
- Snacks (salted chips, nuts, popcorn, pretzels; party dips and spreads).
- Soy meat substitutes.

Tips on Decreasing Sodium and Increasing Potassium Intake

To decrease sodium intake:

- Limit your intake of salty foods.
- Use herbs and spices instead of salt for flavor.
- Use garlic or onion powder rather than garlic or onion salt as a flavoring.

- Decrease salt in your favorite recipes to half or, better, a quarter of the amount suggested.
- Try to add less than ½ teaspoon of salt to your food daily.
- Do not automatically salt cooking water. Use a bay leaf for flavor instead.
- Search for low-sodium or reduced sodium processed foods that are marketed by several companies.

To increase potassium intake, eat more potassium-rich foods:

- All fruits (not just bananas and oranges).
- Fresh and frozen vegetables (without sauces, to avoid added salt).
- Grains, particularly those prepared with little or no salt (like oatmeal, rice, noodles).
- Legumes (dried peas, beans, lentils).
- Unsalted nuts and seeds.

To help reduce your chances of getting high blood pressure, you may wish to decrease your sodium and increase your potassium intake. You will be surprised at the subtle flavors you will notice in foods after you have reduced your salt intake.

Calcium and Phosphorus

It appears that our phosphorus intake has risen in proportion to our decreased calcium intake during the past century. This is because our intake of phosphorus-rich animal protein, soft drinks, and processed foods has increased, while our intake of calcium-rich milk products and leafy green vegetables has decreased. This change in calcium-to-phosphorus balance may be one important reason for the recent appearance of osteoporosis in increasingly younger people. Historically, it has been a disease of the elderly.

Osteoporosis is a condition characterized by a decreased mineralization of the bones. This condition is four times more common in women than it is in men. Estimates indicate that as many as one in every four postmenopausal women has this condition.

Surveys indicate that a minimum of one in every 10 women over the age of 50 suffers from bone cell loss severe enough to cause hip, vertebral, or long-bone fractures.

Besides the calcium-to-phosphorus ratio in the diet, other factors can either speed up or delay the development of osteoporosis. For example, regular exercise and adequate vitamin D intake encourage mineralization of the bones. For more help in protecting your bones from osteoporosis, follow these tips:

Tips on Protecting Your Bones

- Be sure to eat calcium-rich foods daily:
    Try to eat/drink daily the servings of milk products recommended in the Daily Food Guide.
    If you can't digest fluid milk well, try natural cheeses like Cheddar or Jack as a substitute. Processed cheeses and cheese spreads are much higher in phosphorus anyway.
    If you can't digest or are allergic to all milk products, the following foods are rich in calcium:
        Leafy green vegetables: Cup for cup, broccoli, collards, dandelion greens, kale, mustard and turnip greens equal milk in calcium content. The calcium in greens like beet greens, chard, and spinach is not well absorbed, but these are still rich in other nutrients.
        Fish with edible bones: mackerel, salmon, sardines, etc.
        Tofu (soybean curd).
- Obtain adequate vitamin D daily.
    Children need 400 IU daily and adults need 200 IU daily.
    Your body can produce this amount daily with exposure of your face and arms to sunlight for 20 to 30 minutes.
    Each cup of vitamin D fortified milk contains 100 IU of vitamin D.
- Decrease your intake of protein-rich foods to the amount recommended in the Daily Food Guide.
- Get regular exercise (preferably no less than four times weekly; every day would be even better).

Anemia and Iron Absorption

The most common form of anemia—particularly among women—observed in this country is caused by iron deficiency. Therefore, eating plenty of iron-rich foods is helpful in preventing anemia. Such foods are found in the protein-rich foods and the leafy green vegetables groups on the Daily Food Guide. Cooking with an iron skillet will also add iron to the diet.

Iron absorption from the diet and/or from supplements is enhanced if meat, fish, poultry, and/or food rich in vitamin C is eaten at the same time as the iron-rich foods.

VITAMIN SUPPLEMENTS

Do you need to take vitamin and/or mineral supplements? If you are healthy and not overly stressed, the answer to this question is no, provided you regularly eat a variety of fresh and unprocessed foods from the Daily Food Guide. However, you may benefit from the extra insurance of a low-potency, well-balanced multiple vitamin and mineral supplement, particularly if you fit into one or more of the following categories:

1. You eat out frequently.
2. You rely on fast foods or highly processed convenience foods much of the time.
3. You frequently snack on high-fat and high-sugar foods.
4. You regularly skip meals.
5. You go on and off diets in an effort to control your weight.
6. You routinely eat very little—

- less than the recommended minimum number of daily servings from each food group in the Daily Food Guide;
- or less than 1,500 calories daily for those at least 11 years of age;
- or less than 1,000 calories daily for those 4 to 10 years of age;
- or less than 900 calories for those 2 to 4 years of age.

7. You have an illness, anemia, injury, or are recovering from any of these.

If you decide to choose a multiple vitamin and mineral supplement be sure that it contains those nutrients that are not usually added back into processed foods, such as vitamin E, vitamin B-6, folic acid, biotin, pantothenic acid, magnesium, zinc, copper. Biotin is actually made by the bacteria in your digestive tract. However, these organisms can be destroyed by antibiotics, and taking a supplement containing biotin is beneficial if you have to rely on antibiotic therapy over a long period of time.

When choosing vitamin and mineral supplements, compare available formulas with the guidelines in Table 7.

Natural foods consist of vitamins and minerals in complex combinations which interact biochemically with each other. Buying bottles of vitamin and mineral supplements containing single nutrients is not wise, because taking a single element upsets the natural balance of nutrients in your diet. Taking too much of one nutrient can increase your need for one or more other nutrients. Also, it's very costly to purchase nutrients individually.

Supplements are most effective when taken with meals, because food aids in their absorption and use by the body. Also, several smaller doses are absorbed more effectively than one large dose of any supplement. Therefore, a multiple vitamin and mineral supplement, with the daily dose broken into two or three tablets, is the most beneficial, provided you can remember to take them.

Be careful of taking extremely large dosages of supplemental vitamins, particularly the oil-soluble vitamins (A, D, E, K, P), which are stored in the body and can reach toxic levels with prolonged heavy use. You should also limit your intake of the trace minerals (iron, zinc, copper, iodine, chromium, and selenium), which can also reach toxic levels with prolonged heavy use.

It is important to recognize that adding supplements to a diet overly rich in coffee, alcohol, sugar, fat, and salt cannot reverse the damage done by ingesting excessive amounts of these foods. Supplements can never take the place of a healthy diet of fresh and unrefined foods.

TABLE 7: Recommended Formulas for Multiple Vitamin and Mineral Supplements (Based on 1980 Recommended Dietary Allowances [RDAs])

Nutrients	Average RDA (1–10 years)	Recommended Formula (1–10 years)	Average RDA (11+ years)	Recommended Formula (11+ years)
vitamin A	1780 IU*	1780 IU*	3000 IU*	3000 IU*
vitamin D	400 IU**	200 IU**	300 IU**	150 IU**
vitamin E	9 IU***	9 IU***	15 IU***	15 IU***
thiamine	0.9 mg	0.9 mg	1.2 mg	1.2 mg
riboflavin	1.1 mg	1.1 mg	1.4 mg	1.4 mg
niacin	12.0 mg	12.0 mg	16.0 mg	16.0 mg
vitamin B-6	1.3 mg	1.3 mg	2.0 mg	2.0 mg
vitamin B-12	2.5 mcg	2.5 mcg	3.0 mcg	3.0 mcg
folic acid	200 mcg	200 mcg	400 mcg	400 mcg
biotin	90 mcg	90 mcg	100-200 mcg	100-200 mcg
pantothenic acid	3-4 mg	3-4 mg	4-7 mg	4-7 mg
vitamin C	45 mg	90 mg	58 mg	116 mg
calcium	800 mg	240 mg	960 mg	320 mg
magnesium	200 mg	150 mg	330 mg	248 mg
iron	12 mg	12 mg	15 mg	15 mg
zinc	10 mg	10 mg	15 mg	15 mg
iodine	93 mcg	93 mcg	150 mcg	150 mcg
copper	1.5-2.0 mg	1.5-2.0 mg	2.0-3.0 mg	2.0-3.0 mg
chromium	33-133 mcg	83 mcg	50-200 mcg	125 mcg
selenium	33-133 mcg	83 mcg	50-200 mcg	125 mcg

*1 IU vitamin A is equivalent to 0.3 mcg retinol; 3.33 IU vitamin A is equivalent to 1 mcg retinol (as preformed vitamin; does not include carotene).

**400 IU vitamin D is equivalent to 10 mcg cholecalciferol.

***1.49 IU vitamin E is equivalent to 1 mg d-alpha-tocopherol.

SUMMARY

Improving your diet is well worth the effort. You will find that the combination of healthier food choices and an increase in exercise will help you shed unwanted pounds. Chances are good that you'll also notice an increased energy level, shinier hair, clearer skin, and more of a sparkle in your eyes. Common problems like constipation, heartburn, and anemia will also be alleviated when you eat the right foods. And there's a very good possibility that you'll also be able to avoid or at least delay the onset of such chronic conditions as heart disease, high blood pressure, diabetes, and cancer.

To enhance your health and to decrease chances of getting diet-related discomforts and diseases, follow the guidelines below:

1. Eat a variety of foods such as whole grains, colorful fruits and vegetables, lean meats, and low-fat milk products in moderate amounts. (See the Daily Food Guide for more details.)

2. Emphasize fresh, unprocessed foods whenever possible. Make your own mashed potatoes rather than adding water to a boxed mix. Enjoy the treat of a fresh orange instead of an instant orange drink. Keep in mind, too, that frozen orange juice is as good as fresh oranges and superior to synthetic orange drinks.

3. Eat only enough food to maintain your ideal body weight. Remember to eat smaller portions more slowly. Eat crunchy and munchy vegetables when you feel hungry.

4. Eat more unrefined carbohydrates like whole wheat bread, oatmeal, potatoes, legumes, and fresh fruits and vegetables.

5. Eat less sugar and other refined sweeteners. Go very easy on sugar foods like cakes, cookies, candy, pies, and soda pop.

6. Use dried beans, peas, and lentils several times a week in place of fatty meats, poultry, and fish.

7. Eat less fat, particularly saturated animal fats from meat, cheese, cream, and pastries.

8. Avoid consuming too much cholesterol from animal foods and eggs cooked in fat.

9. If you drink alcohol and coffee, do so in moderate amounts.

10. Consume salt and salty foods like hot dogs, pickles, and canned soups sparingly.

Remember, a slow and steady change in the right direction is what counts. It's what you eat 80 percent of the time that's important! Progress slowly and easily into the diet outlined in this chapter, and you will greatly improve both your health and your quality of life.

You have already taken the Life Management Self-Evaluation Test following Chapter 1. Now review the nutrition section, which is repeated here, and see how much you think you can improve your score during the next year by following the suggestions that you've just read for changing your diet.

RECOMMENDED READING

Nutrition and Health

Farquhar, John. *The American Way of Life Need Not Be Hazardous to Your Health*. New York: W. W. Norton & Co., 1979. 195 pages, $4.95.

Ferguson, James. *Habits, Not Diets*. Palo Alto, Cal.: Bull Publishing Co., 1978. 252 pages, $7.95.

Ferguson, James, and Taylor, C. *A Change for Heart: Your Family and the Food You Eat*. Palo Alto, Cal.: Bull Publishing Co., 1978. 183 pages, $5.95.

Mahoney, Michael, and Mahoney, Kathryn. *Permanent Weight Control: A Total Solution to the Dieter's Dilemma*. New York: W. W. Norton & Co., 1976. 192 pages, $13.95.

U.S. Senate Committee on Nutrition and Human Needs. *Dietary Goals for the United States*. 2nd ed. Stock No. 052-070-04376-8. Washington, D.C.: Government Printing Office, 1977. 84 pp., $4.00.

U.S. Department of Agriculture & U.S. Department of Health and Human Services. *Nutrition and Your Health—Dietary Guide-*

lines for Americans. Home and Garden Bulletin No. 232. Washington, D.C.: Government Printing Office, 1980. 20 pages, free.

Wurtman, Judith. *Eating Your Way Through Life.* New York: Raven Press, 1979. 231 pages, $10.50.

Nutrition and Health with Recipes

Cumming, Candy, and Newman, Vicky. *Eater's Guide: Nutrition Basics for Busy People.* Englewood Cliffs, N.J.: Spectrum (Prentice-Hall), 1981. 192 pages, $5.95.

Dinaburg, Kathy, and Akel, D'Ann. *Nutrition Survival Kit.* New York: Jove Publications, 1978. 284 pages, $1.75.

Goldbeck, Nikki, and Goldbeck, David. *The Supermarket Handbook.* New York: Signet Books (New American Library), 1976. 460 pages, $2.95.

Robertson, Laurel; Flinders, Carol; and Godfrey, Bronwen. *Laurel's Kitchen: A Handbook for Vegetarian Cooking and Nutrition.* Petaluma, Cal.: Nilgiri Press, 1976. 508 pages, $18.00 (hardcover). New York: Bantam Books, 1978. 641 pages, $4.50 (paperback).

Recipes Only

Dosti, Rose; Kidushim, Deborah; and Wolke, Mark. *Light Style: The New American Cuisine.* New York: Harper & Row, 1979. 310 pages, $12.95.

Guerard, Michael. *Cuisine Minceur.* New York: William Morrow & Co., 1976. 314 pages, $12.95.

Jones, Jeanne. *Diet for a Happy Heart.* San Francisco: 101 Productions, 1981. 192 pages, $6.95.

Winston, Mary, and Eshelman, Ruthe. *The American Heart Association Cookbook.* New York: Ballantine Books, 1980. 403 pages, $7.95.

My Nutrition

	Points
I feel I overeat:	
Usually	0
Occasionally	1
Rarely	3
I have indigestion:	
Often	0
Occasionally	1
Rarely	3
At the table, I salt my food:	
Usually	0
Occasionally	1
Rarely	3
My refined sugar and sweet food consumption is:	
Average or above	0
Less than average	1
Very low	3
My daily sugar substitute servings are:	
Three or more	0
One or two	1
None	3
My daily alcohol consumption is:	
Three or more drinks	0
Two	1
One	2
None	3
My total weekly egg consumption in all food is:	
Ten or more	0
Eight or nine	1
Seven or less	3

	Points
My bread consumption consists of:	
White	0
Light brown/wheat	1
Whole wheat	3
My cereal consumption consists of:	
Boxed cereals, presweetened	0
Vitamin enriched (with extra roughage)	1
Whole grain	3
My daily soft drink (8 oz.) consumption is:	
Three or more	0
One or two	1
None	3
My daily tea consumption is:	
Five or more cups	0
Two to four cups	1
Two cups or less (or herbal tea)	3
My daily coffee consumption is:	
Four or more cups	0
Two or three cups	1
Decaffeinated	2
One cup or less	3
I use:	
Butter	0
Soft or liquid margarine (or none)	3
My daily roughage intake consists of:	
Normal diet	0
Extra salad and raw vegetables	1
Extra source of fiber once or twice a day	3

	Points
Meat in my diet consists mainly of:	
Fatty meats (untrimmed marbled beef, bacon, luncheon meats)	0
Meats (lean beef and pork, veal; chicken, turkey, and fish cooked with skin)	1
Lean meats (fish, chicken, turkey cooked without skin)	3
No meat at all	3
The dairy products in my diet are mostly:	
Whole milk/cream products (include most cheeses) or imitation dairy products or coconut oil	0
Low-fat dairy products	1
Skim milk or no dairy products, low-fat cheeses, low-fat yogurt	3

My nutrition score is _____

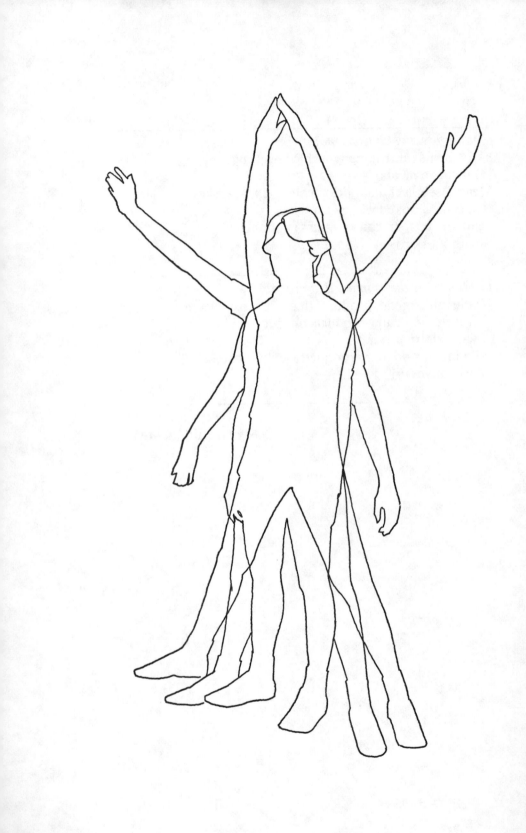

3

Physical Fitness

"Life is movement," wrote a 19th-century European physical training expert. Nearly 100 years ago he hit close to the truth, because physical exercise circulates the most precious ingredient of human life—oxygen—in far greater amounts than when the body is sedentary.

In order to live, each of your body's cells must have constant access to oxygen. Your heart and lungs pump oxygen into the bloodstream, which carries it to all parts of your body. How effectively your cardiorespiratory (heart-lung) system transports oxygen to every tissue of your body is, according to physiologists, the most important measure of your physical fitness.

Your cardiorespiratory efficiency is referred to as your *aerobic capacity*. The easiest way to improve your aerobic capacity is to exercise regularly (at least 30 minutes four to six times a week). Exercise also makes you look and feel better, improves the quality of your sleep and play, helps you cope efficiently with stress, and may ward off—even prevent—serious diseases.

One of the best measures of your physical fitness is your heart rate, because an efficient heart beats more slowly than one that's not fit. A fit person's resting pulse rate is generally in the range of 50–65 beats per minute, while an average person's is 72. Tennis champion Bjorn Borg's resting pulse rate is under 35 beats per minute, which is an indication of the superb efficiency of his cardiorespiratory system. Such low pulse rates are not uncommon among professional athletes and well-trained distance runners.

Let's take a look right now at your own resting pulse rate. You can feel your pulse rate rather easily by pressing your fingers against your temple at the side of your head, or by holding your wrist as you've seen doctors and nurses do.

If you are measuring your pulse rate during or immediately after exercise, count your heartbeats for only 10 seconds and multiply by 6 to get the number per minute. You must take a pulse evaluation following exercise, because your pulse rate slows dramatically as soon as you stop exercising. Studies show that with practice you can become very accurate in taking your own pulse during rest or following exercise. However, it is most important to be consistent and to use the same procedure every time.

An unfit heart must beat 20–30 percent more often than a fit one does, both at rest and while working. In one day it takes more than 25,000 extra beats; in one year an unfit heart beats unnecessarily more than 10 million times. Eventually, because of such chronic overwork and increasing loss of efficiency, your heart, vascular system, and lungs can wear out.

A heart attack is simply the failure of your cardiorespiratory system to deliver oxygen where it is needed, in this case to the heart muscle itself. A stroke is a failure of the body to deliver oxygen to the brain. Many other diseases are also related at least in part to a decreasing supply of oxygen to the body's tissues over a period of many years.

Cardiorespiratory efficiency decreases when arteries and veins become clogged with fatty deposits or when the heart is so overworked and unfit that it pumps out a lower volume of blood. This can contribute to high blood pressure, a second very important measure of your cardiorespiratory efficiency.

It's a good idea to have your family physician take your blood pressure occasionally. A blood pressure reading below 140/90 is considered acceptable and in the normal range. If you do suffer from hypertension, you may be able to lower your blood pressure gradually through regular exercise, body weight reduction, and limited intake of table salt and other high-sodium foods.

Nature didn't intend our bodies to be as sedentary as they have become since we changed from an agricultural to an industrial economy in the 20th century. Our bodies were made to move, to work vigorously as we planted, harvested, and gathered food; tended farm animals; chopped and carried firewood; or walked several miles to visit a neighbor.

In the late 1800s this physical activity was a regular part of everyday life. In modern life, by contrast, relatively few physical demands are made on the body, so we must make a conscious effort to exercise to achieve and maintain physical fitness. That is why exercise has become so important to us in the 1980s—it's the only way we can achieve lifetime health, activity, and physical mobility.

In terms of your health and longevity, cardiorespiratory fitness is supremely important when compared to other components of physical fitness, such as strength and flexibility. At least 80 percent of your physical fitness efforts should eventually be directed toward aerobic activity, which improves cardiorespiratory fitness. You should also seek, however, to achieve a certain level of muscular strength and endurance, as well as muscle and joint flexibility, if you wish to achieve optimum physical fitness and health.

Most people who avoid exercise like the plague do so because they think that exercise is drudgery. It's *not!* Instead, it is tension-releasing fun. It is so enjoyable to exercise, in fact, that large numbers of men and women become positively "addicted" to recreational physical activity every day.

Your watchwords as you begin exercising should be *slow, progressive,* and *enjoyable.* Always do less exercise at first than you feel you can do, because this will keep you from overdoing it. Pushing too hard and making your muscles sore will turn any type of physical activity into drudgery, which will cause you to quickly abandon your exercise program. So *take it easy.*

Begin small and work up very slowly in all physical activities. Work out at least 4 times weekly (the more the better). Start with just 10–15 minutes of exercise, then gradually increase the time (about 2 minutes weekly) until you reach at least 30 minutes of continuous exercise.

In the balance of this chapter you will find numerous tips on how to break slowly into exercising, as well as how to make exercise fun and enjoyable. It's *very* important that you should enjoy exercise if it is to become a lasting part of your lifestyle.

HOW AMERICANS EXERCISE

If you could see graphically how others exercise, perhaps you would find clues to choosing your own personal physical activities. And you *should* choose to do more than one form of exercise. The more variety of physical fitness activities you can include in a regular program of exercise, the greater the interest level over a period of time.

The number of participants keeps growing each year as more people realize the wonderful benefits of exercise. For you, it need not be expensive, because for regular, healthy exercise, we need very little equipment. Clothes to suit the weather and a good pair of walking/jogging shoes will fill the bill.

Physical fitness has become a more than $15 billion-per-year industry, because so many men and women have become vitally interested in their own health and fitness.

Millions of men and women run or jog regularly. Reliable statistics indicate that more than half of us walk on a regular basis, either to work and to do errands or as a planned and relaxing physical activity.

Significant numbers play tennis, bicycle, lift weights, swim, regularly attend aerobic exercise classes, roller skate, ski, play squash and racquetball, golf, or play softball and baseball. While exercise fads come and go, these activities seem to have been confirmed as favorite ways of achieving and maintaining physical fitness. This is not to say, however, that you should by any means be restricted by this list. Literally *any* physical activity that significantly elevates your pulse rate will lead to greater health and physical fitness *if* it's done regularly.

AEROBIC EXERCISE

The relative importance of aerobic exercise has already been mentioned. But what *is* aerobic exercise?

In terms of energy expenditure, aerobic exercise will cause you little or no physical distress. *Aerobic* derives from a Greek word meaning *with oxygen*. So true aerobic exercise is of low intensity and doesn't burn up oxygen quickly enough to make you breathless while you exercise.

Aerobic exercise is also normally carried out for at least 30 minutes. This is because scientists have discovered that exercise results in physical fitness most efficiently if the pulse rate is accelerated during a workout to at least 120–150 beats per minute and kept there for a minimum of 30 minutes. Of course, at first 10–15 minutes will be your starting time-in-action, and you should progress at the 2 minutes per week rate until the continuous 30-minute level is reached.

There are innumerable forms of aerobic exercise. Some of the most enjoyable and most popular are walking, dancing, jogging or running, bicycling, mountain hiking, swimming, rowing, using a mini trampoline, playing a racquet sport (tennis, squash, or racquetball), stationary bicycling, playing handball, downhill and cross-country skiing, playing a team sport (basketball, soccer, baseball, softball, touch football, hockey, or lacrosse), taking aerobic exercise classes, jogging in place, and jumping rope.

Aerobic exercise conditions and improves the efficiency of the heart, vascular system, and lungs. But before commencing an exercise program, men and women over 30 years of age who have been physically inactive for more than two or three years should be sure to have a thorough physical examination. And everyone over 35 should also have an EKG (electrocardiogram) stress test with his or her physical exam. From the results of a checkup, your doctor can discover potential physical problems and accordingly recommend adjustments in the intensity of your exercise program.

The importance of taking a comprehensive physical examination prior to beginning a regular exercise program cannot be stressed enough. Heart, vascular, pulmonary, and other physical irregularities begin to appear for many men and women in their early twenties, and many people are oblivious to such life-threatening problems. For your own safety have your physician check for these ills and then recommend a physical fitness program appropriate for your body. Such a safety procedure might actually save your life.

Aerobic exercise circulates life-giving oxygen in greater-than-normal quantities to all the body's cells, and it burns up significant numbers of calories. Aerobic exercise also temporarily elevates the body's metabolism, so you will continue to burn off body fat faster than usual for several hours after you cease aerobic activity.

How many calories can you actually burn with aerobic exercise? This depends directly on how hard you work to expend energy. The accompanying Table 8 shows how many calories various types of aerobic activity burn in 30 minutes of continuous exercise. This information may also help you choose the types of exercise you will eventually include in your physical fitness program.

Especially when initiating a physical fitness program, it's important to avoid the more strenuous activities, which burn up the greatest number of calories. Ideally, you should keep your pulse rate at a steady state between 120 and 150 beats per minute during aerobic exercise. This heartbeat frequency will yield maximal benefits with minimal physical discomfort.

If you push too hard in a workout and allow your heart rate to exceed 150 beats per minute, you will have exceeded your body's aerobic capacity and you will place yourself in what we call *oxygen debt*. By consuming more oxygen than your body can supply, you are exercising *anaerobically,* the term used to denote strenuous exercise that burns up huge quantities of oxygen.

Exercising anaerobically builds up an oxygen debt, a condition in which the body is actually depleted of its normal oxygen stores. Such an oxygen debt is very painful to endure, and it eventually

Table 8: Calories Expended with Aerobic Activity

Activity	Calories Per Minute
Archery	2.8
Badminton (singles)	6.0
Basketball	12.0
Bowling	3.2
Canoeing (15-minute mile)	7.0
Card playing	1.8
Carpet cleaning	3.5
Cleaning	4.2
Climbing hills	9.5
(with 10-pound load)	10.1
Cooking	3.5
Cross-country skiing	14.0
Cycling (5-minute mile)	10.6
Dancing	
ballroom	5.4
disco	7.5
Drawing (standing)	1.8
Eating	1.7
Field hockey	9.0
Food shopping	4.5
Gardening	3.8
raking	5.4
Golf (foursome—cart)	3.8
Golf (foursome—carrying the clubs)	6.0
Gymnastics	4.6
Handball	10.9
Horseback riding (trot)	8.0
Ironing	2.7

Activity	Calories Per Minute
Jogging (8-minute mile)	12.6
Judo	12.0
Knitting/sewing	1.8
Lying at ease	1.5
Mopping floor	4.8
Mountain climbing	9.5
Music playing (piano)	3.2
Paddleball	10.7
Planting seedlings	4.8
Racquetball	10.7
Roller skating	11.2
Rope skipping (80 turns per minute)	11.3
Running (6-minute mile)	16.2
Scrubbing floors	12.0
Sitting quietly	1.7
Skin diving	12.0
Soccer	12.0
Social dancing	6.0
Softball or baseball	7.2
Square and round dancing	7.0
Squash	10.7
Standing quietly	1.7
Swimming (50 yards per min.)	9.1
Table tennis	5.6
Tennis (singles)	6.0
Tennis (doubles)	4.0
Tetherball	4.6
Trampolining	5.6
Typing	1.8
Volleyball (6 players)	3.6
Volleyball (2 players)	9.2
Walking (17-minute mile)	5.4

© Carnation Company. Used by permission.

forces you to slow down the pace of your workout or stop it alto-
gether.

Here are some comments and recommendations about various
forms of aerobic exercise, including both the positive and the
negative aspects of each type.

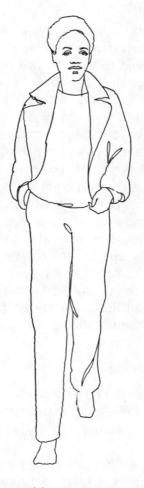

Walking

The least strenuous way to add exercise to your daily routine is
to increase the amount of walking you do. It's a cliche that we hop
into our cars to drive two blocks to the grocery store to buy a loaf

of bread. As long as you have full use of your legs, you can easily walk the two blocks to the market and the two blocks back home with your loaf of bread. And your body will benefit significantly from even this small amount of additional exercise, as long as you do it regularly.

To illustrate the value of regular walking, as well as the ease with which a walking program can be initiated, let's assume, for example, that you are a university administrator who has developed cardiac insufficiency due to long-term physical inactivity. Whenever you need to visit the rest room, walk up one flight of stairs to the one on the floor above your office. This small amount of added exercise is a good starting point.

Then, with time, you can begin to walk up two flights and gradually to walk more around campus. Slowly and easily you can become an inveterate walker, which will reduce your level of useless body fat, lower your pulse rate, and reduce your blood pressure. These are considerable—and possibly life-saving—improvements in your physical condition.

Regardless of how out-of-shape you might be, you should easily be able to walk 10–15 minutes at a slow pace several days a week, gradually working up to as much as an hour of pleasurable, stress-reducing walking. You'll enjoy yourself while walking, you can often work out solutions to your daily problems while on your walk, and your cardiorespiratory system efficiency will be greatly improved by frequent walking.

Jogging and Running

Running is merely a faster form of jogging, in which the participant takes longer strides. The two terms, however, are often used interchangeably. Running, per se, is far more physically demanding than jogging.

From regular walking, it is easy to progress to a program of slow jogging and eventually to running. After several weeks of walking sessions, you can easily and enjoyably begin to intersperse one or two minutes of light jogging with two or three minutes of walking to recover physically from the greater exertion of jogging. Gradually you can do more jogging and less walking, until your entire exercise session consists of continuous jogging for at least 10–30 minutes.

Inexperienced joggers often suffer injuries because they take no precautions against the jarring shock that each foot, ankle, knee, and hip endures when the feet hit the ground—and they do so thousands of times during each exercise session. The best precaution against such injuries is to buy and wear commonly used walking/jogging shoes. Competition in today's athletic shoes has created a generation of excellent shoes for all sports functions.

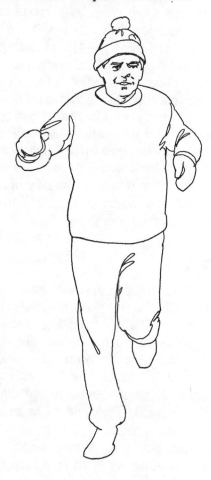

It is also unwise to jog or run on a slanted surface, such as on the side of a roadway, because this puts unbalanced and unnatural strains on your legs and feet, leading to other types of injuries. For the same reason, never jog or run on a rutted field, because that type of uneven surface can also cause abrupt injury-inducing strains on your legs.

Even with new running shoes it is best to keep your running surfaces to dirt, grass, hard sand, or running tracks. Running on roads or sidewalks is all right if these kinds of surfaces are used for less than half the workout. This limit refers only to running and jogging, because all surfaces are acceptable for walking.

If you jog, start out and do it regularly for the minimum amount of time (10–15 minutes), then progress at the recommended increase of 2 minutes per week.

It's always a good idea to take one day off from running each week to allow your body to relax and build up its energy capacity. You should also take time off from jogging or running for at least two or three days whenever you feel any pain in your feet or legs.

Jogging in place offers slightly less aerobic potential than actual running, but the risk of injury is reduced. The main problem with this exercise is that it quickly becomes boring. Still, it may be a nice change of pace on occasion, particularly if it is too cold or wet to jog outdoors.

Bicycling

For many men and women, bicycling is a more enjoyable form of aerobic activity than walking or running. Bicycling is much easier on the feet and legs than running. Most of the body's weight is supported by the bicycle seat, which minimizes orthopedic strain on the lower extremities (hips, legs, ankles, feet).

Build up your total riding mileage on a bike as gradually as you might increase your total amount of running. You should also ride on marked bicycle paths rather than on well-traveled roadways, since the risk of an automobile-bicycle accident is nil when you are riding on a bike path. To be safe, however, be sure to wear a helmet when you are bicycling.

As a general rule, bicycling two miles is approximately equivalent aerobically to walking or running one mile.

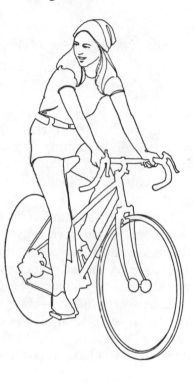

Stationary Bicycling

Many men and women enjoy pedaling a stationary bike while watching television or when the weather is inclement. Obviously, there is little, if any, risk of injury while riding a stationary bicycle, and the degree of aerobic conditioning you can achieve using one is quite high.

Swimming

Swimming is even easier on your body orthopedically than bicycling, because the water buoys up the entire body. Unfortunately, many individuals do not have ready access to swimming pools or other swimming facilities.

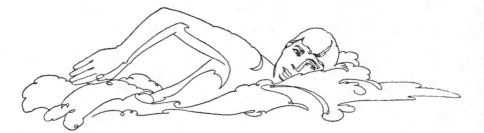

It makes little difference what stroke you use while swimming, because all swimming strokes stimulate the cardiorespiratory system quite efficiently. For the sake of variety and greater enjoyment, you can easily alternate strokes every one or two laps of the pool.

The key to swimming is relaxation. Most novice swimmers thrash and fight their way through the water, needlessly tiring themselves and severely limiting the distance they can swim without stopping to rest. Experienced swimmers, in contrast, seem to glide efficiently and almost effortlessly through the water.

Consistent practice—always concentrating on staying relaxed as you swim—will soon turn swimming into an enjoyable experience for you. You may also benefit from a private lesson or two, particularly if you have a flaw in your swimming technique.

Racquet Sports

All racquet sports—tennis, badminton, squash, racquetball, and, for our purposes, handball—are similar in their aerobic effect on the body and their potential to cause injury. The stop-and-go action of racquet sports *can* become anaerobic, but the player may be oblivious to the oxygen debt because of the intense concentration required to follow the flying and/or bouncing object of play.

The quick stops and starts inherent in racquet sports can put severe stress on all of the leg joints, particularly the ankles. These stresses occur less frequently than in ordinary running but are of greater severity. So the leg injury potential inherent in racquet

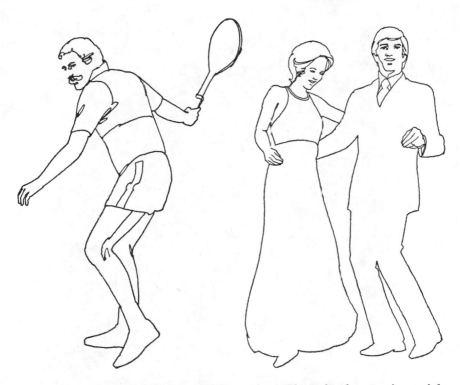

sports is slightly higher than in running. There is also a minor risk of eye injury in most of these sports, so many participants wear protective equipment over their eyes.

Dancing

If you enjoy music and social contact, you will find dancing one of the most enjoyable of all aerobic activities. And if you are self-conscious, a few inexpensive dance lessons will quickly alleviate this problem. Most individuals who refuse to dance do so simply because they don't know how to do it.

Ballet, jazz, and modern dance classes, as well as social dancing, are highly enjoyable ways to achieve excellent aerobic fitness and a superior degree of body flexibility. Dance training also develops a grace of movement and elegance of body carriage unattainable through other exercise.

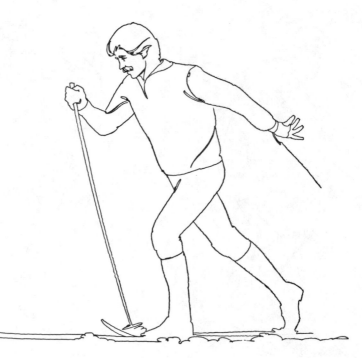

Skiing

Skiing is an excellent activity. Cross-country skiing offers superb aerobic exercise. Downhill skiing is fun; however, it requires greater skill, practice, and training, and it is less of an aerobic activity.

Cross-country skiing can burn more calories than downhill skiing. Moreover, there is a potential for injury in downhill skiing that is not present in cross-country skiing. If you decide to do considerable downhill skiing, you should undertake a serious preconditioning program. Far more injuries occur during the last run of the day, when the body is too fatigued to adjust quickly to an unexpected mogul or rough spot in the snow. By being sure you are fully conditioned before going on the slopes, you can drastically reduce the risk of injury. The best preseason ski conditioning program would consist of at least one month of weight training on the program outlined later in this chapter. You should also practice daily the stretching program outlined in this chapter, as well as spend at least 15 minutes a day in aerobic activity. This combined conditioning program will greatly reduce the risk of injury on the slopes.

Cross-country skiing is quite safe, and it offers a much higher degree of aerobic conditioning than downhill skiing if it is practiced regularly. Among competitive athletes, cross-country skiers consistently have the most efficient cardiorespiratory systems.

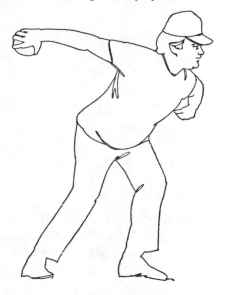

Team Sports

The accent throughout this chapter has been on improving physical fitness in the most enjoyable manner possible, and team sports are favorite ways to enjoyably seek physical fitness. Twice as many men and women participate regularly in the team sports of softball, baseball, volleyball, touch football, basketball, soccer, and lacrosse combined than in any other physical activity. Many people find it easier to physically express themselves by participation in a team sport than by taking a solitary jog. Moreover, team sports give you the advantage of improving your endurance and strength, as well as helping to tune up your cardiovascular system.

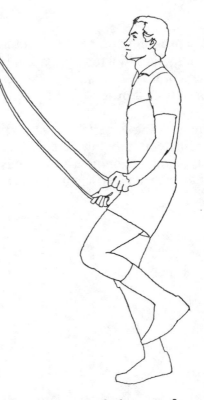

Jumping Rope

Jumping rope can be another good change of pace when out-door exercise is impossible. The potential for developing aerobic conditioning through jumping rope can vary widely, according to how high, how fast, and how long you jump. For variety, you can practice double turns (turning the rope twice on one jump) or crossing your hands in front of your body when jumping rope. In addition to the aerobic benefits of jumping rope, you will find this activity tones and strengthens all the muscles of the legs, particularly those of the calves.

Other Activities

Numerous other activities have minor potentials for increasing aerobic conditioning, but they should still not be overlooked if you enjoy doing them. Some of these are golf (if you don't ride a cart), bowling, weight training, and gardening.

Integrating Aerobic Exercises—The Total Program

You will be most likely to retain interest in and enthusiasm for an aerobic exercise program if it includes a wide variety of physical activities. You can easily walk a few minutes each day simply by walking at times when you would ordinarily drive your car a few blocks to do an errand. Or you can walk up two or three flights of stairs when you could have taken an elevator.

Then, at other times of the day, you can alternate aerobic workout sessions of running, bicycling, swimming, dancing, skiing, hiking in the mountains, participating in a team sport, or playing a racquet sport. Regardless of the activity, your heart and lungs will benefit greatly from it, as long as you do aerobic workouts several days a week and gradually increase the duration and intensity of each exercise session.

As an example, here is a relatively strenuous program containing six to eight aerobic exercises per week for beginning and intermediate male and female participants:

Monday	Tuesday	Wednesday
Walk to work	Bicycle to work	Walk to work
or	or	or
Swim 15–30 minutes	Play racquetball	Run ½ mile

Thursday	Friday	Saturday
Bicycle to work	Walk to work	Bicycle 5–10 miles
or	or	or
Walk ½ mile	Dance	Play tennis

This is, of course, only a sample program. You should adjust your individual program to your unique energy level and also include in it those aerobic activities that you enjoy participating in the most.

STRETCHING AND FLEXIBILITY

While flexibility training is less important than aerobic exercise in terms of your general health and physical fitness, it still is an important component of all-around physical fitness. Significantly, there are no limits on the age of those who can benefit from a stretching program. Senior citizens and individuals with serious injuries can often still stretch when orthopedic problems prevent them from doing other forms of exercise.

There are seven basic reasons for adopting a stretching program:

1. It improves your health and fitness.
2. It improves your physical appearance.
3. It prevents injuries.
4. It improves athletic performance.
5. It is a good warm-up/warm-down for other types of training.
6. It improves body mobility.
7. It can be enjoyable.

You would benefit most from doing stretching exercises 8–10 minutes just before beginning your aerobics program.

How you stretch is vitally important. When stretching correctly you should slowly ease into the stretched position until you begin to feel that the muscle is stretched tight. Back off one or two degrees from this maximum stress position and hold that position for 10–15 seconds (often called "required length of time") before relaxing the stretch. Later, as you grow more fit and ambitious, you can do a second and third repetition of stretching exercises.

Never bounce into a stretched position. You can very easily injure yourself while stretching "ballistically" like this, and you will receive far less benefit from bouncing and forcing a stretch than from one done in a slower and more relaxed manner.

Your Stretching Exercises

Begin by doing each of these stretches in the order listed, for only a few seconds. Then gradually work up to the point where you are doing each stretch for 10–20 seconds. Two or three 10–20 second stretches should get the job done.

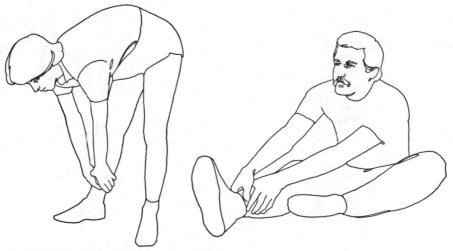

1. Standing Hamstring Stretch

Stand erect and place your feet 2½–3 feet apart with your toes pointed slightly outward. Extend your arms directly downward. Reach toward your right ankle with your hands. Grasp your ankle. Keeping your legs straight throughout the stretch, gently pull your torso toward your right ankle until you reach the maximum stretch for 10–15 seconds. Relax the stretch just enough to avoid extreme discomfort and hold the stretch for 20–60 seconds. Relax and repeat the stretch on the other side. This movement stretches the hamstring muscles at the back of your thighs and your lower back muscles.

2. Hurdler's Stretch

Sit on the floor or on an exercise mat. Extend your right leg directly forward and hold it straight throughout the exercise. Place the toes of your left foot against your right thigh as high up your leg as possible. Rest the outside of your bent left leg on the floor. From this position, lean forward and grasp your right ankle with both hands. Gently pull your torso down toward your ankle until you reach the maximum stretch possible without forcing it. Back off a notch and hold this position. Repeat the movement with your left leg extended forward. The hurdler's stretch stretches your hamstring, groin, lower back, and upper back muscles.

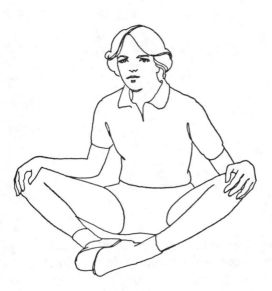

3. Seated Groin Stretch

Sit on the floor or on an exercise mat and extend your legs outward at 45-degree angles from your body. Bend your legs and place the soles of your feet together. This movement will force you to raise your knees up off the floor. Pull your feet as close to your crotch as you comfortably can. Then use your hands to press down on your knees until you feel the stretch of the muscles of your hip girdle. Back off a notch from this maximum stretch and hold that position. This movement stretches all the muscles in and around your pelvic structure.

4. Standing Thigh Stretch

Place your left hand on the back of a chair, on a tabletop, or on any other solid object to balance your body in position during this stretch. Bend your right leg fully and reach back with your right hand to grasp the toes or ankle of your right foot with your right hand. From this position, pull up on your foot until you feel the muscles on the front of your right thigh reaching the maximum stretch level. Retreat a little from this level and hold that stretched

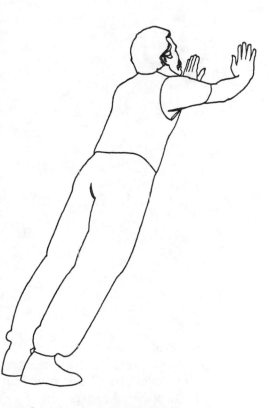

position. This movement stretches the muscles at the front of your thigh as well as in the lower part of your frontal abdomen. Repeat exercise with left leg and left hand.

5. Calf Stretch

For this exercise you will need to face a wall. Stand 2½–3 feet from the wall and place your hands on it at about shoulder height (your fingers should be pointed upward). Place your feet at about shoulder width and be sure your toes are pointed straight ahead. Stiffen your body. From this position, try to force your heels down to the floor. If you can do this comfortably, simply walk your feet backward another half step and repeat the movement. Calf stretches will soon make the calf muscles and Achilles tendon at the back of your lower legs much more flexible.

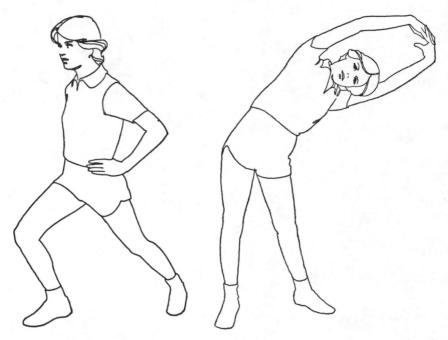

6. Lunging Stretch
Stand erect with your feet shoulder width apart and your toes pointed directly ahead. Place your hands on your hips and hold them there throughout the movement. From this starting position, step 2½–3 feet forward on your left foot. Keeping your right leg as straight as possible, fully bend your left leg. At the bottom of the movement your torso should be upright. Your right leg should be straight, and your right knee will be two to three inches from the floor. Your left leg will be fully bent, and your left knee will be at least three to five inches ahead of your left ankle. Hold this stretched position for the required length of time. Repeat the movement with your right foot forward. This exercise stretches the frontal thigh muscles on the back leg and the buttocks and hamstring muscles on the back of the front leg.

7. Side Bend Stretch
Stand erect and place your feet slightly farther apart than shoulder width. Your toes should be pointed either directly ahead

or slightly outward. Extend your arms directly overhead and clasp your hands. Keep your arms and legs straight throughout the movement. From this position, bend as far to the right side as is comfortable and hold that stretched position. Repeat the movement to the left side. This type of stretch makes the muscles along the sides of your waist and torso more flexible.

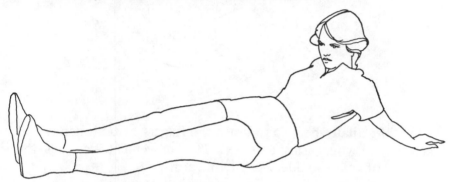

8. Lying Chest/Shoulder Stretch

Sit on the floor or on an exercise mat and extend your legs outward, directly in front of your body. Keeping your arms straight, place your hands flat on the floor at shoulder width as far behind your body as possible (your fingers should be pointed to the rear). Then slowly slide your hands farther and farther to the rear until you reach the maximum stretch for the muscles of your shoulders and chest. Back off a couple of degrees and hold this stretched position for the required number of seconds. This exercise stretches the muscles of your chest and shoulders as well as your biceps muscles to a smaller degree.

9. Seated Arm and Shoulder Stretch

Sit on the floor or on an exercise mat and fold your legs into a comfortable position. Extend your left arm directly upward. Then, leaving your upper arm motionless, bend your left elbow and extend the fingers of your left hand directly down your back. At the same time, fully bend your right arm and reach upward along your back with the fingers of your right hand, trying to touch the fingers of your left hand. As you grow more flexible,

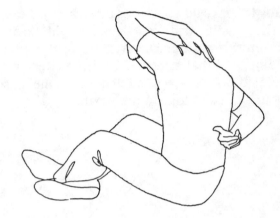

you will actually be able to grasp the fingers of both hands and gently pull your arms together. This movement stretches the muscles of your shoulders, chest, and arms.

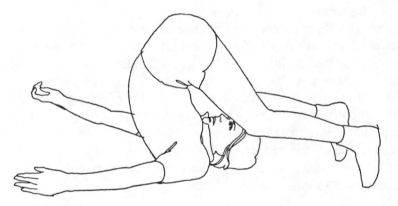

10. Lower Back Stretch

Lie on your back on the floor or on an exercise mat. Extend your body and place your arms straight along the sides of your torso. Press your arms to the floor or mat and raise your legs upward until your knees are above your face. Bend your legs and try to touch your knees to the mat or floor at the sides of your head. Hold this stretched position for the required number of seconds. This exercise efficiently stretches the lower back and hip muscles.

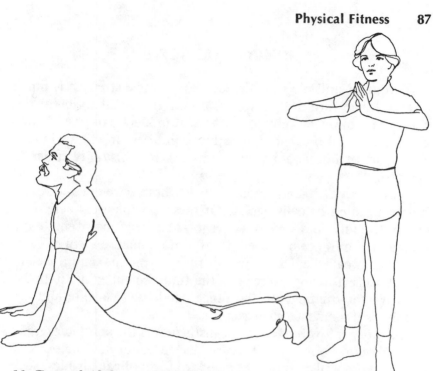

11. Frontal Abdomen Stretch

Lie face down on the floor or an exercise mat. Place your hands on the floor by the sides of your shoulders (your fingers should be pointed forward). Keeping your legs and hips in contact with the floor or mat, push your shoulders up off the mat as high as you can. Hold this stretched position for the required length of time. This movement stretches the muscles along the front of your abdomen.

12. Hands-Wrists Stretch

Stand erect with your feet a comfortable distance apart. Place your fingertips and thumb tips together directly in front of your chest, elevating your elbows so the upper arms are parallel to the floor. Then push the heels of your hands toward each other until you reach the maximum stretch in your fingers and/or wrists. Back off on your stretch and hold this stretched position for the required number of seconds. This exercise stretches both your fingers and wrists.

MUSCLE STRENGTH

In your overall physical fitness plan, muscle strength is much less vital than cardiorespiratory fitness, but it's still an important component of overall physical fitness. A moderate degree of muscle strength will prevent many athletic injuries. It will also make every sort of household chore and work responsibility easier to perform.

Muscle strength and endurance are best developed through weight training or calisthenics. Of these two physical activities, weight training does a much better job of developing strength and muscular endurance because it is a far more intense form of exercise than is calisthenics. With calisthenics, the maximum weight you can use for any exercise is the total weight of your body. With weight training, on the other hand, you can literally use hundreds of pounds in each exercise.

The most enjoyable form of calisthenics is the aerobic exercise class. Several books have been published about aerobic exercise programs, as well as about the standard form of calisthenics, such as sit-ups, push-ups, and knee bends.

Even though more than 15 million men and women train with weights, many millions more avoid weight training because they have been misinformed about the activity. Weight training need not make your muscles tight, slow you down, injure your back, make a woman look like a man, or build the large muscles of a bodybuilder. It can greatly strengthen all the muscles of your body, however, and it allows you to selectively build up skinny parts of your body or reduce fatty areas.

The most common form of weight training is done with barbells and dumbbells. Barbells are merely steel bars of various lengths on which are fastened flat, pancake-like metal discs that allow one to increase or decrease the weight on the bars; barbells are generally about five feet in length, while dumbbells are shorter versions of barbells, 12–14 inches long. Dumbbells are held in one hand (most commonly one is held in each hand).

Numerous weight training machines also are available in schools, health spas, YMCAs, and other locations. Overall, machines are safer and more easy to use than are free weights (barbells, dumbbells, and other related equipment).

Generally speaking, you can receive nine major benefits from a weight training program that takes no more than 30–40 minutes per day, three days a week:

1. Improved physical fitness.
2. Greater muscle strength and endurance.
3. The ability to shape and sculpture your body.
4. Improved overall health.
5. Greatly and quickly improved sports performance.
6. Relief from the tensions of everyday life.
7. Improved muscle and joint flexibility.
8. A more positive self-image and greater self-confidence.
9. A new physical activity that can easily be shared with friends, spouses, and families.

The easiest way to initiate a regular program of weight training is to join a health spa or gymnasium. These are listed in the yellow pages, and virtually all such facilities will offer competent instruction and supervision.

Your Weight Training Program

A general weight training program for beginners (those with less than six weeks of weight training experience) is given in Table 9 on the following page. It is recommended that if weight training is a new form of exercise for you, you should discuss such a program with your physician beforehand. That way, you will know whether your back and other areas of your body are ready for these exercises. This program can be performed using only an inexpensive barbell and a flat, narrow bench. The program should be undertaken on three nonconsecutive days per week—e.g., Mondays, Wednesdays, and Fridays. You should do 8–12 repetitions (counts) of each set (grouping of repetitions) for each exercise. You should rest for 60–90 seconds between sets. Once you can comfortably do 12 repetitions of an exercise, add several pounds to your barbell and drop back to doing eight repetitions, then work up gradually again to doing 12 repetitions.

TABLE 9: Weight Training Program

Exercise	Sets	Repetitions	Men	Women
1. Sit-ups	1	20–30	0	0
2. Deadlift	2	8–12	40	25
3. Squat	3	8–12	40	25
4. Barbell Bent Rowing	3	8–12	40	25
5. Bench Press	3	8–12	40	25
6. Upright Rowing	2	8–12	35	20
7. Military Press	2	8–12	35	20
8. Barbell Curl	2	8–12	35	20
9. Barbell Wrist Curl	2	12–15	40	25
10. Standing Calf Raise	3	15–20	50	35

A suggested starting weight for men is listed under the column marked "Men," and the suggested women's starting weight is listed in the "Women" column. When calculating this poundage or weight, be sure to include the total weight of your barbell. Add the weight of both of the discs to the weight of the bar (calculate the weight of the bar by multiplying each foot of the bar by 5 pounds).

Initially you may find weight training to be a more strenuous physical activity than anything else you have ever tried. If you attempt to do a full workout the first time you train with a barbell, your muscles will become very sore. To prevent this, do only one set of each exercise for your first workout. During the next week add a set to each exercise requiring two or three sets. Finally, at the beginning of the third week you may safely do the whole program. Do not, however, attempt to add weight to any exercise before you finish your slow, gradual break-in of the full program.

Do each set of every exercise before moving on to the next movement. Breathe out rhythmically on the raising phase (cycle) of each exercise and breathe in as you lower the weight. When you are doing bench presses, always make sure to have a safety spotter on hand to rescue you should you fail to push the weight up to arm's length.

Exercise Descriptions

By carefully comparing the drawings of each exercise with the following descriptions, you can learn to do each weight training exercise safely and without additional coaching.

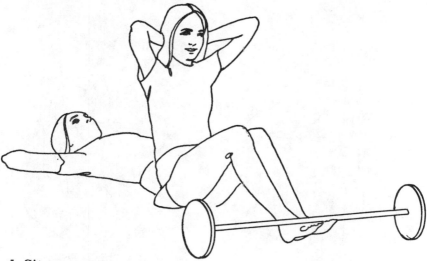

1. Sit-ups

Lie on your back on the floor and slip your toes under a couch or other heavy piece of furniture. Bend your knees approximately 30 degrees to take potential strain off your lower back as you do your sit-ups. Place your hands behind your neck and hold them in that position throughout the movement. From this basic starting position, simply curl up slowly until your torso is perpendicular to the floor. Return to the starting point and repeat the movement. Sit-ups develop the muscles of your abdomen (stomach).

2. Deadlift

Stand up next to a barbell that is lying on the floor. You should be close enough to it so your shins touch the handle of the barbell. Bend over and take a shoulder-width grip on the barbell so your palms are facing your legs. Bend your knees and dip your hips so your knees are below your hips and your shoulders are above your hips. From this position, and keeping your arms straight through-

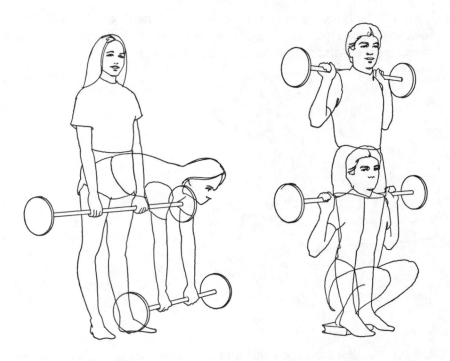

out the movement, simultaneously straighten your legs and back to stand erect with the weight dangling at straight arm's length across your upper thighs. Return the weight to the starting position and repeat the movement for the required number of repetitions. Deadlifts develop the muscles of your lower back, your thighs, and your hips.

3. Squat
Place a barbell across your shoulders and behind your neck, balancing it in position by grasping the barbell bar out near the plates. Place your feet at shoulder width and angle your toes outward approximately 45 degrees on each side. Keeping your torso as upright as possible, slowly squat down until your thighs are parallel to the floor. Be sure as you squat that your knees travel outward at 45-degree angles over your feet. Do not bounce at the

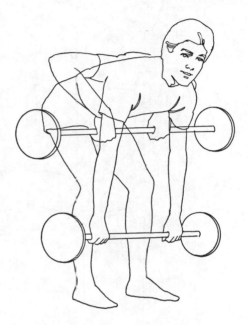

bottom of the movement. Slowly straighten your legs and return to the starting point. Squats strongly stress the muscles on the fronts of your thighs, your hips, your buttocks, and your lower back. If you have difficulty squatting flat-footed, stand with your heels resting on a two-by-four-inch board or book when you do squats.

4. Barbell Bent Rowing

Grip the barbell as for the deadlifts but let your arms hang down straight with your torso parallel to the floor and your knees slightly bent. The barbell should be hanging at arm's length, directly below your shoulder joints and clear of the floor. Maintaining this body position, pull the barbell straight up to your chest. Lower it back to the starting point and repeat the movement. Barbell bent rowing works all of the muscles of your upper back, plus the muscles of your biceps and forearms.

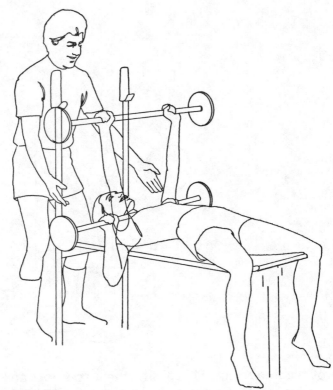

5. Bench Press

Again grasp the barbell with the same grip as for the deadlift, then lie back on a flat exercise bench. Extend your arms directly above your chest, so that they are perpendicular to the floor. From this position simply bend your arms slowly and lower the barbell straight downward until it touches your chest. Push it back to the starting point and repeat the movement. Bench presses strengthen the muscles of your chest, shoulders, and triceps.

6. Upright Rowing

Stand erect with a barbell in your hands and your arms hanging straight down (the barbell will be resting across your upper thighs). You should have a narrow grip on the barbell (no more than six inches between your index fingers), and your palms should be facing your body. Keeping your body stiffly erect, bend

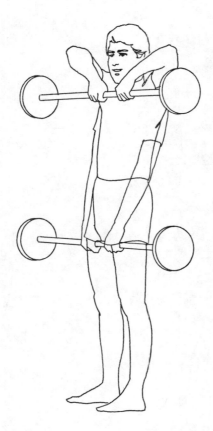

your arms and slowly pull the weight upward, close to your body, until it touches the underside of your chin. Throughout the movement your elbows should be held higher than your hands. Lower the weight slowly back to the starting point and repeat the movement. Upright rowing strengthens the muscles of your shoulders, upper back, and arms. It is also an excellent movement for promoting good shoulder posture.

7. Military Press
Take the same grip on a barbell as for deadlifts. Pull the barbell up to your shoulders so it rests across your upper chest and move your elbows directly under the bar. Stand erect throughout the

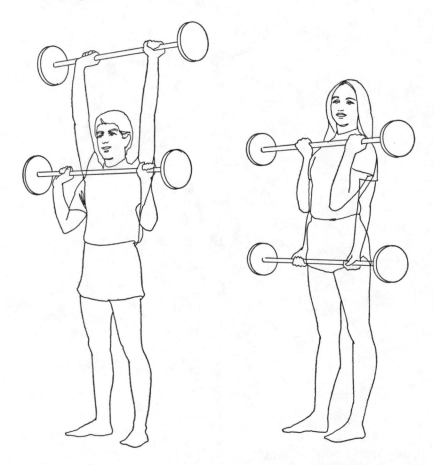

movement. Starting from this position, slowly push the barbell directly upward until it is at arm's length above your head. Lower the weight back to your shoulders and repeat the movement. Military presses strengthen your shoulder and triceps muscles.

8. Barbell Curl

Stand erect with a barbell in your hands, your arms hanging straight down with the barbell resting across your upper thighs. You should have a shoulder-width grip on the barbell, your palms should be facing away from your body, and your arms must be straight at the start. Keeping your body motionless and your upper arms pressed against your sides, bend your arms and slowly move the barbell in a semicircle from your thighs to your chin. Lower the weight back down along the same arc to the starting point and repeat the movement. Barbell curls develop the muscles of your biceps and forearms.

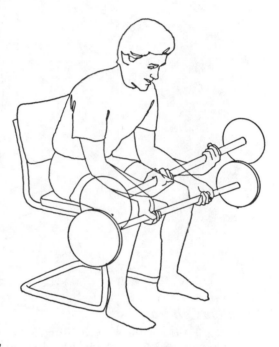

9. Barbell Wrist Curl
Take the same grip on a barbell as for barbell curls. Then sit at the end of a flat exercise bench or a chair and place your feet on the floor at shoulder width. Run your forearms along the tops of your thighs so your hands and wrists hang off the edges of your knees. Your palms should face upward. Then sag your wrists downward as far as you can. From this starting position, use your forearm strength to curl the barbell upward in a tight semicircle as high as you can. Return the weight back along the same arc to the starting point and repeat the movement. Barbell wrist curls develop the muscles of your forearms and strengthen your grip for racquetball, tennis, and all other sports.

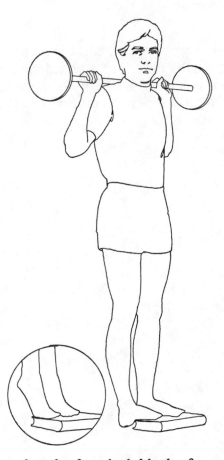

10. Standing Calf Raise

You will need a thick book or a four-by-four-inch block of wood
to do this movement best. Place a barbell across your shoulders as
if preparing for a squat. Then place your toes and the balls of
your feet on the book or block of wood. Your feet should be 8–10
inches apart on the block. With successive sets you can point your
toes directly ahead, angle them inward at 45 degrees on each side,
or angle them outward at 45 degrees on each side. Each toe position stresses different aspects of the calf muscle. From this starting position, and while keeping your legs straight, slowly rise up
as high as you can on your toes. Slowly lower back to the starting
point and repeat the movement for the required number of repetitions. Standing calf raises develop all of the muscles of your lower
legs.

A COMPLETE FITNESS PROGRAM

Anyone with at least partial use of his or her legs and arms should exercise. Age makes absolutely no difference as long as the spirit is willing and you progressively increase the intensity of an exercise program gradually and slowly. You should also be willing to exercise regularly.

Almost everyone has been in poor physical condition at one time or another, and if you are in such condition, the prospect of exercising regularly can be abhorrent. But you must believe that from your very first low intensity exercise session, you will begin to feel better and enjoy life more. And you'll soon discover that the act of exercising itself can be supremely pleasurable.

Begin your program of physical rejuvenation with light aerobic activity every other day. Then, as you gradually and comfortably rebuild your physical fitness, you can progressively increase the frequency and intensity of your aerobic workouts. But be sure to make every workout fun; otherwise, there's little sense in exercising. Pushing hard enough to make your workouts painful will very quickly cause you to abandon them.

You should include stretching exercises in your physical fitness plan, even if your program consists of only walking and light jogging. The best way to include stretching is to use your flexibility workout as a warm-up to any form of aerobic activity or strength training. Such a stretching warm-up will reduce the chance of injury in any other type of physical activity.

Within another month, if you feel so inclined, you can initiate some type of strength training program two or three days per week. Again, weight training will develop muscle strength much more quickly than calisthenics will, but the choice is up to you. Pick whichever mode of strength training you find most enjoyable.

To review, every man and woman who adopts a program of regular exercise can expect to reap five major benefits:

1. You will develop a more efficient cardiorespiratory system, thereby strengthening your heart, lungs, and vascular system, and increasing your body's ability to transport and utilize oxygen.

2. You can control your body fat far more effectively and look more lean and attractive for the rest of your life.

3. You can make stress work for you instead of against you.

4. You will increase your muscle strength, endurance, and flexibility, which can prevent low back pain and retard the general physical decline due to disuse that often comes with aging.

5. You will perform all tasks—especially of the person-to-person type—with greater alertness and clarity because exercise-increased blood circulation is stimulating. You will experience an improved sense of well-being.

You won't receive these benefits overnight, since you can't rebuild your own physical fitness in a day or a week. But once you have succeeded in rebuilding your fitness, you will experience an indescribable sense of self-satisfaction.

TEST YOURSELF

In Chapter 1 you took the Life Management Self-Evaluation Test. Now review the physical fitness section, repeated here, to see how much you think you can improve your score in the next year by using what you have learned in this chapter. Set a reasonable goal to work toward—and get started.

My Exercise, Occupation, Recreation, and General Fitness

Activities	*Points*
My exercise program consists of:	
Little or no exercise	0
Walking program three or more days per week	1
Easy to moderate exercise three or more days per week	2
Fairly vigorous exercise in exercise attire three or more days per week	5

	Points
Heavy exercise in exercise attire three or four days per week	8
Heavy exercise in exercise attire five to seven days per week	10

My occupational activities consist of:

Mostly mental activity with little or no manual labor	0
Combination of mental and manual labor	2
Mostly manual labor (I perspire from my work)	4

My recreational activities and hobbies consist of:

Gardening, doubles tennis, sailing, reading, and other sedentary activities	0
Singles tennis, hiking, light bicycling and other moderately fatiguing activities	2
Prolonged and fatiguing physical activities	4

Activities score _____

Weight

The average person in good physical condition reaches a desirable weight between the ages of 18 and 23. Comparing your weight then and now, you are presently:

10	9	7	5	2	0	-2	-4	-6	-8	-10
At or below that weight	1-3 lbs. over	4-6 over	7-10 over	11-15 over	16-20 over	21-30 over	31-40 over	41-50 over	51-75 over	76 or more over

If you have always been overweight, circle how many pounds overweight you now are.

Weight score _____

Systolic blood pressure

	-5	-3	-2	-1	1	4	6	7	8	9	10
Male	180	160	150	140	135	130	125	121	118	115	110
Female, premenopause	177	157	147	137	132	127	122	119	116	113	108
Female, postmenopause	184	164	154	144	139	134	129	125	122	118	113

If not known, check here _____ and circle 4.

Systolic score _____

Diastolic blood pressure

	−5	−3	−2	−1	1	4	6	7	8	9	10
Male	99	96	93	90	88	84	80	75	70	68	65
Female, premenopause	99	95	90	88	86	83	78	73	68	66	63
Female, postmenopause	99	97	95	92	88	86	82	76	73	68	65

If not known, check here _____ and circle 4.

Diastolic score _____

My total fitness score is _____

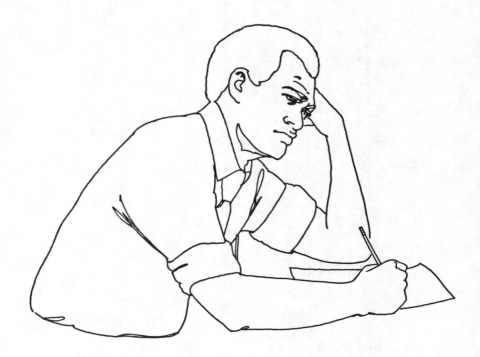

4

Reducing Stress

At its most fundamental level, stress is any demand placed on the human mind and body.

Stress affects all of us—regardless of our age, sex, or occupation—and it may be either good or bad. Stress, however, is generally thought of as a negative force that attacks all of us who are living in today's nonstop, high-pressure society.

The world's foremost authority on stress is Hans Selye, an Austrian-born physician who conducts his research at the University of Montreal. Dr. Selye has written, "You should not and cannot avoid stress, because to eliminate it completely would mean to destroy life itself. If you make no more demands on your body, you are dead."

So stress is a physiologic response to all experience. The body responds to stress-producing situations, or stressors, with a series of changes in body chemistry—glandular reactions that result in sudden increases in pulse rate, blood pressure, and blood sugar—and these in turn initiate resisting or compensating bodily responses. Dr. Selye called the process the "adaptation response" and found that continued exposure to stressors that cause significant responses could cause the resistance to wear down or become exhausted. This, in turn, creates a need for relief to avoid harmful or lasting effects. In this chapter you will learn how to identify the stressors in your life and bring those that are most harmful under control.

Subjected to the most extreme form of negative stress, your body will respond with what has been called the *fight or flight syndrome*. Under such conditions men and women are capable of performing unbelievable physical tasks. As an example, a middle-aged, 110-pound Florida woman was able to lift the front end of a Cadillac high enough to free her son who had been pinned under the car when a jack slipped.

Such an extreme physiological reaction to stress occurs only in life-threatening situations. Perhaps at some point in your life you have perceived yourself to have been in danger, such as when walking at night in a strange neighborhood. In such a situation, the mind perceives stress and this almost instantly leads to an outpouring of the powerful hormone adrenalin from the adrenal glands into the bloodstream.

Immediately, adrenalin significantly increases your heart rate and respiration rate, elevates your blood pressure, and causes your skeletal muscles to ready themselves for sudden and powerful contraction. It also simultaneously activates vital organs such as the liver and deactivates other unnecessary organs and systems such as the digestive system. Thus, as a result of the fight or flight syndrome, the body is fully prepared to fend off impending death by either standing and fighting, or by turning and fleeing.

In modern society—although we still have this primitive defense mechanism built into our bodies—we are seldom faced with life or death situations, so our physiological stress mechanism usually reacts to a far lesser degree. Still, it does respond to the negative physical and mental pressures that we perceive, and in doing so it ultimately can harm the body.

Our own stressors are usually rather mundane when compared to a caveman fighting a saber-toothed tiger, but they do build up and accumulate significant burdens on our stress-response mechanism. The degree to which we are stressed multiplies with the complexity of our lives.

Virtually everything we do each day in our complex society—from driving home in teeth-clenching rush-hour traffic to listening to a recitation of all the world's problems on the 6 o'clock news—produces at least small amounts of stress. To remain in optimum health we must learn to cope with stress.

In his book *The Stress of Life,* Dr. Selye reveals that the chronic presence of stress-related hormones in the body eventually reduces its ability to resist disease. The immunological system actually begins to wear out, and we become vulnerable to a wide range of diseases. Some researchers even believe that cancer can be induced by unmanaged stress.

The human body simply can't be expected to respond constantly to heavy negative stress stimuli without having its blood pressure and heart rate remain dangerously high. And this is precisely what takes place within the bodies of individuals subjected to heavy daily stress. Eventually the hypertension or elevated pulse rate, or perhaps even negative psychological effects resulting from long-term heavy stress, causes the body to break down. This may not happen to you, but you may already exhibit other, less profound symptoms of stress-related physical or mental disorder. Here is a comprehensive list of symptoms that can be associated with stress-related illness:

- Grinding the teeth (particularly while sleeping)
- Migraine or tension-induced headaches
- Increased smoking
- Increased alcohol or drug use
- Insomnia, fitful sleeping, nightmares
- Irritability
- Depression
- Anxiety
- Shoulder, neck, or back pain
- Sexual dysfunction
- Chronic fatigue

- Indigestion, heartburn
- Hypertension, elevated heart rate
- Irregular pulse rate (a racing pulse)
- Skin eruptions, skin dryness
- Spontaneous sweating
- Overeating or undereating
- Poor concentration, learning disability
- Frequent flu or colds
- Persistent body infections
- Loss of enjoyment of life, apathy
- Lack of physical coordination
- Skipped menstrual periods or irregular cycles
- Impulsive, irrational behavior
- Thyroid dysfunction
- Forgetfulness
- Unexplainable pain
- Speech problems (stuttering, slurred speech)
- Dependence on tranquilizers

If you exhibit one or more of these symptoms, you may need to try to identify and neutralize the stressors.

RECOGNIZING YOUR STRESSORS

Very few individuals will have difficulty identifying those stressors serious enough in their lives to require attention. Some of the most familiar stress situations include difficulty with an employer or coworker, an unfulfilling romance, a sickly or unhappy child, long lines at the bank or grocery store, car problems, unfriendly or noisy neighbors. Stress may be caused by such everyday events as missing a train or bus, not receiving an expected salary increase, being given unreasonable work deadlines, falling short of achieving a personal goal, being served by a surly waiter, or receiving unexpectedly high bills.

Any time you feel pressured by someone or something, you are under stress. That's the easiest way to identify your stressors. Over a period of a few days you should be able to observe and

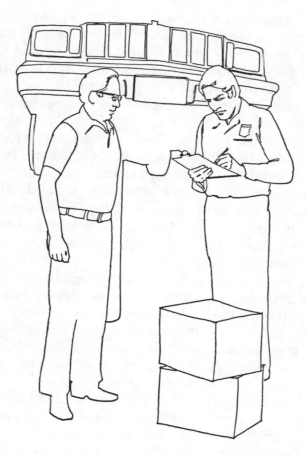

identify your major stressors. It will be helpful to make a mental
or written note of each so you can work on reducing their effects.

Most commonly, stress will be found at work, in family and
personal relationships, and in social situations. A frequently en-
countered example of work stress is an overload of assignments.
Let's assume that you take a new job and soon find yourself over-
loaded with projects. You complete each one as quickly and efficiently as possible, but gradually you fall behind. This pressurized
situation continues for several months with no feedback from
your employer.

Abruptly, two of your projects are sent back to you with your employer's extensive instructions for reworking. As soon as you resubmit those two projects, you are invited to lunch with your employer, not by him personally, but by his secretary. Uncertainty magnifies the stress bearing down on you. Is your employer displeased with your work? Will you be terminated? Or is the luncheon meeting merely a belated personal welcome to the company?

Regardless of the outcome, your stress level will be high until the uncertainty is resolved. Change is as stressful as uncertainty.

There are several ways to deal with these types of job stress, and each of these methods will be discussed in greater detail later in this chapter. For instance, you can manage such stress through sharing your experience with close friends, by hard and distracting exercise, use of various relaxation techniques, or in many cases by the final resolution of the problem.

Another example of job stress could be working on a monotonous assembly line. The monotony can be stressful by itself, but even more could be the loss of personal identity when working at such a job. This type of stress can be relieved most efficiently by achieving personal recognition. By playing on the company softball team, or serving on a safety committee, you might quickly notice a diminishment in your stress levels.

Regardless of the stressor in any depersonalizing situation, you can help solve the problem by finding something you are good at to occupy yourself and establish your self-identity. Actors paint, executives may play golf or fish. Excelling at something brings self-satisfaction, and hence relief from stress.

The break-up of a long-term relationship is a tremendously stressful situation. Growing friction in a relationship can also be enormously stressful. In these situations, professional counseling can be most helpful. Many companies offer counseling in employee assistance programs; some people seek help with personal problems from family doctors, hospital-based psychologists, or clergymen. Encounter groups can help to establish a base in an apparently friendless situation. The effectiveness of such groups is not so much a function of the ability of the leader, but of the interaction established by the group.

Many men and women find it difficult to meet new individuals and make friends in social situations. In reality, fears of meeting new people and worrying about what they will think of you are largely unfounded, but those who are troubled may be helped by practicing conversational skills with friends or relatives, and gradually building up a circle of new friends.

THE AGE FACTOR AND STRESS

Certain types of stress are unique to specific age groups. For younger children the most devastating form of stress is lack of love and affection. Even the youngest child has a very acute perception of this.

Undoubtedly children may also undergo great stress from the perception of a rocky parental bond, or, ultimately, a broken marriage. The divorce rate is rampant, and it is having a devastating effect on the children of parents who are divorcing or divorced. In broken families, the best recourse for the child or children is the understanding love of both parents, and, especially, the one who is with the children most of the time.

The best antistressor for children is a strong and healthy family life laced liberally with love. With "family medicine" like this, most children are able to adapt to their outside environments with ease.

As children grow up and assume more and more responsibility, stress can escalate. Being free to succeed or fail totally on one's own merits can be very stressful. The suicide rate in any society is directly related to the level of stress. You might be surprised to know that suicide is now the second leading cause of death (after accidents) among men and women under 20 years of age.

Again, a strong and supportive family is the best solution to helping a teenager cope with the growing stresses he or she perceives.

Later in life, decision-making becomes a stressor. There are hundreds of life-forming decisions that must be made by each individual, a few of them of seemingly supreme impact. Decision-making should be approached in a relaxed and nonmechanical way. Delay making an immediate decision if you feel it will produce stress. Spend time researching the possible consequences of a decision, writing down all the variables. Ask the opinions of others whom you trust and who have greater knowledge and experience than you do.

Stress is related to the self-perception of one's contribution to society, so this type of stress increases with age. The elderly are often despondent because they feel that they have no worth to anyone anymore.

A sensitive family environment is as important to the elderly as it is to children. Those who nurtured should eventually nurture again. With imagination, the children of aging parents can innovate ways in which to include their parents in family decision-making and the care of grandchildren. Elderly men and women whose families are not near enough for visiting may avoid stress by living with or near others of their generation or joining social groups at churches, community houses, or senior centers.

THE EASY WAY OUT

You shouldn't automatically attack your stress-related problems with medication, as millions of Americans are doing today. Many medications may actually cause more stress than they relieve, and, at best, drugs may mask the symptoms without getting at the cause.

Unless they are prescribed by a physician who is familiar with you and your problems, instead of resorting to drugs to cope with stress, you should attack your stress-related problems with self-knowledge, common sense, persistence, and determination. This is the safest and most natural method of managing stress.

HOW TO COPE WITH STRESS

The easiest way to cope with some stressors is to simply run away from them. It's easy enough to avoid minor stressors by easing yourself out of stressful situations when you can, but this isn't solving any problems. It's difficult and often impossible to move to a more congenial neighborhood, for example, and usually even more difficult to change jobs. While you can literally run away from some of your stressors, most of them are so deeply woven into the fabric of your life that they are simply unavoidable. In such cases your only recourse is to do everything in your power to minimize their effects.

Regular Exercise

One of the best methods of coping with stress is to maintain a program of regular exercise. Exercise dissipates life's tensions efficiently. After a long and stressful day, nothing seems to feel as good or dissipate stress so thoroughly as building up a sweat participating in some type of strenuous physical activity. And along with that physical well-being, you will have the satisfaction of knowing that you have accomplished something worthwhile toward improving your health and building a healthier lifestyle. Both results are effective ways to relax and relieve stress.

Actually, stress studies have shown that exercise causes the brain to release a hormone called *endorphin,* which many researchers consider a natural opiate. It elevates your mood without harmful side effects and without a noticeable "crash" after the effects of endorphin wear off. So whenever you hear someone talking about "getting high on exercise," you'll understand what's meant.

Relaxation Techniques

There are numerous ways to relax and minimize the effects of stress on your mind and body. One of the easiest ways to relax is to concentrate on and control your breathing patterns. Lie in a comfortable position on your back on the floor or on your bed. Place a pillow under the backs of your knees and another one under your head. Lay your arms at your sides in a natural position, perhaps bending them slightly, and place your palms flat on the floor or bed.

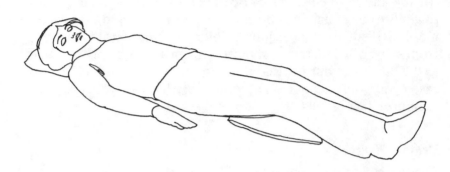

Once or twice per day when you feel stressed, spend 10 minutes in this position, breathing slowly in and out. Inhale deeply while slowly counting to four, hold your breath for a count of two, and exhale slowly while again counting to four. Concentrate *only* on this slow, deep breathing.

Don't actually time yourself while you are breathing under such full control and concentration. Think only of breathing in and out, and within 5 to 10 minutes you will find that you are completely relaxed. You may even feel as though you are floating in space. Lie there for a few minutes, savoring this stress-free condition, and then get up and go about your daily tasks again. When you feel overstressed again, repeat this breath-control technique.

Another type of relaxation can also be practiced in this same supine position. Start this technique with four or five minutes of breathing control, until you are fairly relaxed. Then begin *thinking* the tension out of your left foot, for example, telling yourself that the tension is draining slowly away and your foot is completely relaxed. In a few seconds it actually *will* be relaxed.

Repeat this process with your right foot. Then slowly work upward in small increments until you have finally relaxed every part of your body, including the muscles of your neck and head. Although it will take longer to accomplish this at first, as you become more adept you will be able to complete this process in only 10–15 minutes. And mastering this technique will give you a profound sense of relaxation.

Once you have relaxed your whole body, again lie there for a few minutes in a state of deep relaxation, fully enjoying the feeling of being totally stress free.

Massage is another good relaxation technique, though it requires the skills of another person. Most health clubs have a masseur or masseuse, and having a full-body massage once or twice a week can be very relaxing.

Relaxing for 10–15 minutes in a hot tub, sauna, or hot bath is another way to reduce stress, and you can use it on an almost-daily basis. Heat is very soothing to the body, which slowly relaxes as a result of it, and eventually your mind goes along with your body and also relaxes, greatly reducing your stress levels.

Meditation

Many people have found meditation techniques helpful in reducing stress. Among the better known methods are Transcendental Meditation, Mantra-Repeating Meditation, Zen Meditation, and Focal Point Meditation (in which one stares hypnotically at an object). You may have a friend with knowledge about one or more of these types of meditation, and he or she can help you to decide if meditation will help reduce your levels of stress. Also, books on meditation can be found in most libraries or bookstores.

Practiced once or twice per day, meditation may greatly reduce your feelings of stress. It can transport you from the place where you are subjected to stress to a fantasy place, or someplace where you were once very happy.

Arguing with Yourself

One interesting stress-reducing technique that psychologists suggest is self-control, which you can think of as arguing with yourself. In this method you simply talk to yourself, telling yourself how trivial a particularly stressful situation really is when compared with something else that has happened to you and which you survived unscathed.

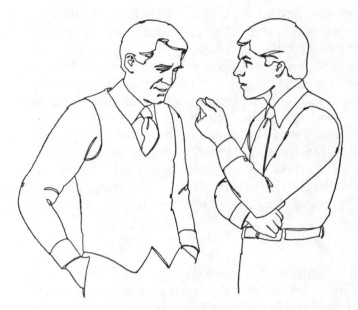

Talking to yourself can be quite effective, because most persons have a tendency to exaggerate their problems. Actually, there are very few really *serious* situations in life. Almost anything can be talked out, either internally or with someone you trust. Then, when your problem has been worked out, your level of stress will go down.

Relying on a Friend

If you have difficulty in arguing out a problem with yourself, try talking about it with a close friend. It is surprising how many stressors you have in common with your friends, and they may already have been through the crisis you are facing. Whether familiar with your situation or not, friends will probably be able to give you a new perspective on your problem. The best person with whom to discuss a problem could be your spouse, clergyman, or someone else you trust in an intimate conversation about your innermost fears and problems.

One popular method of brainstorming a problem is to get on the phone and talk to several of your friends or relatives. With a wide variety of opinions, you have a broad base from which to attack your stressor.

Hobbies

Stress experts recommend that overly stressed individuals adopt hobbies to disengage themselves from the manic pace of life. Any type of recreational activity—and the more physically demanding it is, the better—will reduce your perception of being overly stressed.

The range of hobbies and recreational activities that you can practice is extremely broad. Choose one that appeals most to you or choose several hobbies or recreational activities that you can practice or escape to on a regular basis. And one of the best of all methods of relaxing and avoiding stress is to join some useful organization or group activity with programs and goals devoted to helping others. The company of worthwhile people, being away from familiar work conditions, and above all the satisfaction of serving your community and its people who need help are unsurpassed means of taking you "out of yourself" and leaving your problems behind.

Diet Factors

Nutrition is definitely a factor in stress reduction. Chronic illness is a leading contributor to stress, and a health-promoting, balanced diet will help you to maintain good health. Reducing your level of body fat will allow you to move about with less effort and participate more fully and fruitfully in recreational activities. Obesity is also a contributing factor in many life-threatening diseases. Moreover, controlling your weight will make you feel better about yourself; you will be less shy, more self-assured—and these qualities contribute substantially to the relief of stress.

When reducing your body weight avoid fad diets, which are often harmful. A simple low-calorie diet and an increase in the frequency and duration of aerobic exercise will gradually and safely reduce your body fat level. (For an idea of your appropriate body weight, refer back to Chapter 1, page 30.)

Reducing your sodium intake (see the suggestions for this procedure in the nutrition chapter) can help reduce your blood pressure, one of the most common symptoms of high stress. One gram of sodium retains 50 grams of water in your body, and excess water retention contributes to high blood pressure.

Overall, diet and exercise are among the most important factors in reducing stress levels, yet they are also among the most neglected of all stress-reduction methods.

BENEFICIAL STRESS

At the beginning of this chapter, Dr. Hans Selye observed, "You should not and cannot avoid stress, because to eliminate it completely would mean to destroy life itself. If you make no more demands on your body, you are dead."

Positive, beneficial stress—the stresses of joyous occasions, challenging tasks, stimulating companionship—can give you confidence and help make life worth living. Such stresses add excitement; without them you would find life boring. Without the self-imposed stress of challenge you would cease to grow as an individual, and would actually exist in a state of stagnation.

With practice, you can condition your mind to use small, self-induced stresses to spur you on to greater accomplishment. As an example, you can set a goal of increasing your work production. This in turn puts more pressure (or stress) on you to succeed. But such self-induced stress is easily accommodated.

Successful and happy persons tend to be goal-oriented. They stress themselves beneficially—but within reasonable limits—by setting higher and higher goals, conditioning their minds to accept each new stress. They reach their goals, and this in turn leads to setting even higher goals, which makes self-induced beneficial stress a constructive force in our lives.

CONCLUSION

Life is full of negative stresses, which can jeopardize your physical and mental health if they are allowed to accumulate. But negative stresses *can* be dealt with and either eliminated or greatly reduced.

By eliminating or reducing negative stress, you can greatly improve your health and fitness lifestyle. Both the quality of your life and your life span can be increased by following the stress management suggestions outlined in this chapter. They work well and can be easily incorporated into your lifestyle, so use them to become healthier and happier.

Repeated here from Chapter 1 is the personality and stress section from the Life Management Self-Evaluation Test. Think about what you can do to change attitudes and relieve stresses in your life. Keep in mind that your job may create stress, which means you can't do much to alter your scores in certain job-related sections of the test. You therefore should try to improve your score in those sections of the test where you have more control over things, such as your emotions and social relationships. Then set a goal you think you can achieve in the next year to improve your health score.

My Personality and How I Handle Stress

	Points
I am anxious/nervous:	
Often	0
Occasionally	1
Seldom	3

	Points
I would describe myself as:	
Highly competitive	0
Moderately competitive	1
Not competitive	3
When confronted with a situation that bothers or angers me:	
I keep it to myself	0
I may or may not say something	1
I always say something about it	3
Criticism or scolding bothers me:	
Greatly	0
Moderately	1
Hardly at all	3
In my work, success is:	
Very important	0
Moderately important	1
Not important	3
I go out of my way to avoid unpleasant acquaintances:	
Often	0
Occasionally	1
Rarely	3
I have spells of the blues:	
Often	0
Occasionally	1
Rarely	3
I have disturbed sleep:	
Often	0
Occasionally	1
Rarely	3
People disappoint me:	
Often	0
Occasionally	1
Rarely	3

	Points
I am depressed:	
Often	0
Occasionally	1
Rarely	3
In my own work, I am confronted with making important decisions:	
Often	0
Occasionally	1
Seldom	3
"Our country is going to the dogs" is a statement with which I:	
Agree greatly	0
Agree moderately	1
Agree hardly at all	3
I am sexually frustrated:	
Often	0
Occasionally	1
Rarely	3
I am secretive:	
Greatly	0
Moderately	1
Hardly at all	3

My personality/stress score is _____

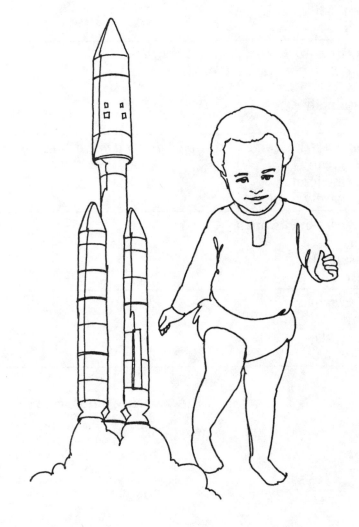

5

Your Health and Fitness Lifestyle

Lasting changes in lifestyle don't occur with the speed of a rocket flight into outer space. Instead, they occur in small and manageable increments, much like a young child's halting and uneven steps. Making meaningful, positive changes in your health and fitness lifestyle—comfortably and enjoyably—may actually take more than a year. But you *can* make positive changes with a little systematically applied effort.

Good health and fitness ultimately depend on you. There are no magic solutions. No pills, chemicals, or other gimmicks can provide you with good health habits. However, by understanding yourself and taking gentle but definite responsibility for change, you can easily and enjoyably develop an improved health and fitness lifestyle.

In the previous three chapters you've read what you need to know about the factors that make up the health and fitness lifestyle. But how do you implement these to achieve a positive, lasting lifestyle?

123

Undoubtedly you've tried to diet or to initiate an exercise program at least once in the past, and then failed to continue it. Perhaps you have failed again and again, so the idea that you can diet, exercise, and control your stresses probably seems impossible. Through moderate behavior modification techniques, persistently and correctly applied, you can move mountains. You can change your bad habits to good ones, effecting a dramatic improvement in your health and fitness lifestyle.

A PLAN OF ACTION

Your habits are patterns of behavior that meet your life needs. Such habits are often essential to your performance and production, but they can also work against you.

While you've spent a lifetime developing habits that make your life workable, not all of your habits meet positive needs. Overeating, lack of exercise, drug usage, excessive drinking, and chronic vocational and family stress are well-documented habitual barriers to good health. For most people, developing an optimum health and fitness lifestyle becomes a matter of simultaneously reducing the number of negative habits and increasing the number of positive habits.

Fortunately, you can adopt certain behavioral principles that will encourage positive habits and discourage negative habits. Like the moderate changes in lifestyle suggested in earlier chapters, these changes can be applied to your everyday life with little effort. Perhaps for this very reason, they seem to work for many people where all previous efforts to change have failed.

Initially, you may think you lack the necessary motivation or self-control to change your habits. The following methods will prove so simple that anyone can succeed with them. The only requisite to successful habit change is your willingness to *try*.

One Step at a Time

Changing your lifestyle can sometimes appear to be such an overwhelming task that it boggles a person's mind. For some odd reason the average person often tries to change his lifestyle all at once. Instead, he should take the same plan of attack in changing his lifestyle as he takes in solving other problems: break it into smaller problems and attack each of them, one at a time.

The ancient Chinese philosopher Confucius had an excellent grasp of this concept when he wrote, "The journey of a thousand miles begins with a single step." The journey can be your total change in health and fitness lifestyle. Similarly, each step along the journey is a smaller problem to be overcome.

You will be most successful in changing your habits if you think in terms of long-term and short-term goals. Your long-term goal is achieving optimum health and fitness (or walking a thousand miles). Your short-term goals should include each step along your thousand-mile journey.

You can have literally thousands of short-term goals, and each of them should be attainable within a few days. As an example, suppose you are working up to running three miles nonstop. There are roughly 5,300 yards in three miles, so you could set short-term goals of 100 yards each. In this case, if you ran 100 yards more each day, it would take you 53 days to reach your goal.

Here's another example of how you might change your lifestyle: Let's assume that you want to lose 2 pounds of fat. One pound of fat consists of 3,500 calories, so to lose 2 pounds you would have to eat 7,000 calories less than normal over a period of time. One pat of butter consists of approximately 100 calories, and it would be very easy to avoid eating one pat of butter per day. Seventy days of avoiding this pat of butter could quite easily result in a 2 pound weight loss.

Each time you reach an intermediate goal, such as running 3 miles or losing 2 pounds (which can be equated to the rest stations along your thousand-mile journey), you should set another, higher goal. Break it into manageable short-range goals and begin working toward each of them.

Over a period of time, hundreds of achieved short-range goals can lead you painlessly to your long-range goal, lifetime health and fitness.

What's the Problem?

The first and most important step toward changing habits is identifying each problem habit in turn. If you are going to assess your health adequately, you must start with the real problem, namely yourself. Look realistically at your own personality. The details of any habit change program you ultimately design must fit your psychological strengths and weaknesses if it is to be successful. Answer these questions:

- Are you more energetic in the morning or in the evening?
- Are you gregarious, or independent?
- Do you look to others or to yourself for the majority of your support?
- How important is it to you to impress others?
- How compulsive are you?
- What do you value most in your life?
- What are some of your favorite rewards for good behavior?
- What reasons have you given yourself in the past for failing to change positively one or more bad health habits?

There's no reason whatsoever for you to compile an exhaustive psychological profile of yourself. But it might help to write a paragraph or two about yourself. Pay particular attention to times of peak energy, your social lifestyle, your problem behavior, and the things that genuinely give you pleasure.

At this point, old-fashioned common sense should begin to help you start building some of the foundations of your habit change program. As an example, if you're overweight and have had difficulty losing body fat on your own, then joining a group weight loss program may make plenty of sense.

You'll also probably see patterns that will influence your exercise habits. If your peak energy levels occur at 4:00 P.M., for example, early morning jogging efforts may be doomed to failure. If you're competitive and like to impress others, team sports may be better for you than jogging or lifting weights alone in your basement. And if you're an organized, success-oriented person, you might find written goals and detailed charts of your weight-reduction or exercise progress to be helpful adjuncts to your plan.

How You Fit In

You should next examine your work and family situation. Answer these questions:

- How much time do you have available to devote to programs of habit change?
- When is that time exclusively yours?
- How might family responsibilities create barriers to change?
- How might work responsibilities affect your program?
- What are you already doing at work or at home that contributes to good health and could be increased without undue effort?

Armed with general information about your own personality, your work, and family situations, the final step of your personal assessment is to complete a detailed analysis of each of the specific problem habits you wish to change. This will be your attempt to look at the events immediately preceding and following an incident of negative behavior in order to determine what is causing and helping you to continue such negative behavior.

Record Your Behavior

Choose one aspect of your health and fitness lifestyle improvement program—nutrition, exercise, or stress management—to work on first. Keep a diary of your behavior in relation to that aspect for at least one week. As an example, let's examine your dietary habits.

Each day write down everything you eat, including the amounts of food consumed and the time that they were eaten. Record where you ate the food—e.g., in a restaurant, in front of the television, at a sporting event, in your dining room, at your desk at the office. Also note your emotions while eating—feelings of depression, illness, fatigue, anxiety, happiness, and so on. Write down names of other people who were present and what happened during the first minute or two after consuming the food or drink.

Next, analyze each class of information in relation to your problem behavior. Look particularly at your feelings before and after you ate. Is your eating behavior related to anger, depression, boredom, or anxiety? Compulsive eating often is caused by failure to distinguish between hunger and other feelings, so any negative emotion can make you want to eat or drink.

An important bonus this analysis provides is that your habits can almost automatically begin to improve once the analysis starts. The act of monitoring or recording food eaten, the number of cigarettes smoked, the amount of alcohol consumed, the chronic stresses in your life, or the number of days without regular exercise almost always leads to an initial positive habit change. Observing your behavior thus becomes the start of self-control. Completing the assessment phase leads naturally to beginning a positive behavioral change.

Getting Started

As you begin to change your health and fitness habits, use your analysis to help create a realistic plan of attack. You must start out knowing that you need to fight the *cause* of each bad habit, not the habit itself. And you needn't be ashamed of occasionally backsliding.

If you were strong and had ironclad motivation and self-control to begin with, you wouldn't now have poor health habits. Taking responsibility for your actions is essential, but it is equally important to develop an attitude of patience with yourself as you change. This is where all the information you've collected about yourself comes in handy, because it allows you to identify and list your weaknesses and those situations where you currently lack self-control.

Your program for change is based on avoiding situations in which you cannot control your problem habits and then slowly and patiently building self-control, day by day. Gently accept your failures and pat yourself on the back for your successes. You

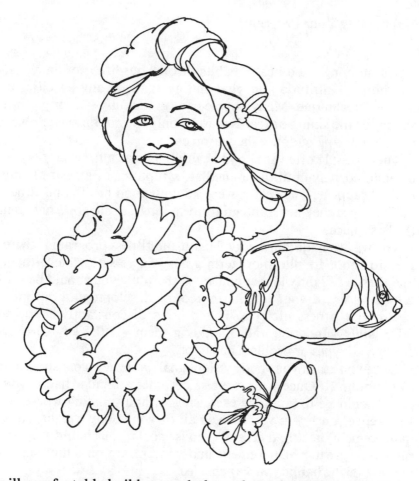

will comfortably build strength through persistence, so that if you do have a bad day you can get right back on the program, and slips don't become program failures.

It also helps to build some immediate rewards into your program. Go back to your analysis and locate the things you find rewarding or of value. Then pick several rewards to give to yourself during the first month of your habit-changing program. Buying a suit of clothes or a new dress to shrink into makes good psychological sense. Putting the money you save on unpurchased liquor or cigarettes into a vacation fund is another good idea.

Maintaining Your Program

Maintaining good health habits throughout life is often a matter more of attitude and goal setting than of any specific behavioral technique. Many people can successfully diet or get into shape for the skiing or tennis season, only to gain the weight back or quit working out once the season ends.

These people often see good health habits as a necessary evil to be endured only until the immediate symptoms of an out-of-tune body disappear. They can never maintain good health and fitness habits, since they never intend to form long-lasting good habits in the first place.

The way to maintain a good health and fitness program is therefore to shoot for the short-term goals you've set, achieve them, and then set slightly higher goals. All the while you should be progressing toward your long-term goal of developing an optimum health and fitness lifestyle. This process of constantly changing your goals—updating and upgrading them—is the key to overcoming all types of problem behavior.

Once you reach your body weight goal, your new goal should be to maintain it. Once your exercise becomes a regular habit, your goal should be to continue exercising without missing workouts. In essence, once you've achieved all of your body weight, stress management, health, diet, and exercise goals, you should stop emphasizing greater achievement and concentrate on simple maintenance of the habits you've achieved.

It also helps to start to focus your attention after four or five months from more external, artificial rewards (such as weight loss) to more intrinsic reinforcements such as the feel of your body in good tune sweating through a workout, the extra spring in your legs, your increased energy levels, or the improved self-esteem resulting from your improved physical appearance or the pure joy of effortless physical movement.

Eventually, good health will become a habit in itself. Your success will start to build on itself. Your workouts won't take as long to complete on a maintenance program, nor will they result in sore

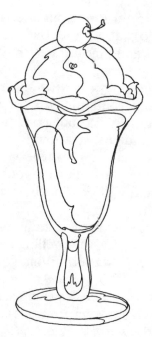

muscles, because you're building on a system that is already in good health.

A final key to maintaining your program is to recognize that we all tend to become bored very easily. So it's important that you vary the types of foods that you eat, the ways in which you manage stress, the type of exercise that you do, and the types of rewards you give yourself for a job well done.

The human mind and body are very adaptable mechanisms and they very quickly cease to adapt to the same external stimuli. But if such stimuli (rewards, foods, types of exercise) are changed frequently, the mind and body are never able to grow accustomed to these stimuli. Therefore, boredom never sets in.

DEALING WITH THE CHALLENGE

An improving lifestyle does feed on itself. As you improve your mental and physical health, the changes in your lifestyle take root and flourish. And, in turn, as your lifestyle improves, so does your health. This is logical, isn't it? But you still must start by improving your mental and physical health. The ways to go about this follow.

1. *Use positive relaxation techniques.* Getting away from your problems by diverting your mind to some other topic usually works, at least temporarily. It's not a bad technique, but don't kid yourself that this is genuine relaxation. It isn't.

Instead take 10–20 minutes, whenever you feel particularly stressed, to lie flat on your back with your legs elevated approximately a foot above the floor. This is intended to be a physical *and* mental maneuver.

Let all of your muscular tension drain out of your body. Sense your slowing heart beat, feel the swelling begin to leave your legs, and experience a flush of warmth filling your head and torso (see page 114).

Only when you are in a state of genuine relaxation can you find the perspective to confront your problems realistically.

2. *Keep your work and play in a healthy balance.* Work goes well with play, and play goes well with work. A balance between the two is very much a part of the wellness lifestyle.

Play can become merely a diversion apart from exercise. Some people play chess in their free time. For others, exercise is synonymous with play. Thus, jogging, bicycling, running, swimming, and weight training become physical fitness "treatments" while simultaneously providing a participant's innate need for play time.

3. *Adopt sensible exercise habits.* Whether or not exercise also becomes play to you, your new lifestyle *must* include a program of regular exercise. Such programs have been discussed in detail in Chapter 3, and you should adapt that information to your needs, personality, and time schedule.

The single most significant lifestyle change over the past century probably has been a dramatic reduction in the total amount of physical activity required in our daily lives. We don't walk; we ride. We don't do farming or manual labor; we work in offices. After a drastically shortened work week, we have gained so much leisure time that we have become weekend sports spectators, deriving satisfaction from *other people's* physical accomplishments.

More than 2,500 years ago, Plato observed that only the strongest and healthiest of bodies is able to withstand the rigors of inactivity. He must have been predicting the sedentary society of the 1980s. Because our normally inactive bodies need physical activity, exercise is probably the most important key to changing your health and fitness lifestyle.

What's so magical about exercise? When you exercise, you begin to feel better about yourself almost immediately. You have more energy, feel stronger, sleep better, are more relaxed, and experience lowered blood pressure and cholesterol levels. You also lose weight, because exercise acts as an extremely effective appetite depressant. Exercise results in a new image of yourself and a new sense of self-worth.

When we view ourselves as energetic, vigorous, healthy, vibrant individuals we tend to resist any temptation (e.g., eating a hot fudge sundae) that would ruin that image. And we eagerly strive to follow any diet or do whatever type of exercise improves the way we look and feel. Any momentum toward wellness develops a snowball effect through which the momentum grows greater and greater by feeding off higher and higher accomplishments.

If a small amount of fitness motivation is followed by a resultant increase in exercise, changes rapidly begin to take place within the body. At first these changes are just physiological adaptations to the effort, but soon these adaptive body changes stimulate further increases in motivation.

The happy result of this cycle is that you can make very significant gains in physical and mental health over a long, gradual period of time, while avoiding pain and suffering. Instead of pain, you will experience considerable self-fulfillment and pleasure.

We've talked about the cornerstones of a wellness lifestyle. Now let's take a quick look at some suggestions that can make changing your lifestyle easier, more satisfying, and considerably more fulfilling to you.

1. Begin to reach for a life free of negative influences. Clear your mind of old pains and negative images and then anticipate

upward mobility. Once you do this, *how to get from here to there* can become a very simple exercise in mental dedication.

2. Work on changing your attitude. Although your health—and, to a great extent, your habits—must evolve, your *attitude* toward life can change much more quickly.

3. Don't make a whipping post of yourself. Self-blame and unwillingness to forgive oneself lie behind every known type of self-abuse.

4. If you are at fault, think first of yourself as someone who is experiencing and learning, not as a person winning or losing. Realize that mistakes are unavoidable and forgive yourself. Take as much time as is necessary to think through and analyze the incident completely. Then get used to the fact that, as a human being, you will frequently make mistakes. Finally, learn from each mistake you make so you can avoid repeating it.

5. Think ahead in providing for yourself. Try napping, then exercising before attending a play, film, or party. Appreciate how this strategy enhances your enjoyment. Be constantly prepared to live life to the fullest.

6. Develop an *observing ego*. To accomplish this, imagine that you are stepping out of yourself to observe your deportment from a distance, objectively yet in a kindly manner.

7. Accept advice if it is directed toward improving your function in any activity that's meaningful to you.

SUMMING UP

Let's now attempt to pull together everything you have been told about developing a new health and fitness lifestyle. The time has come to make meaningful and positive changes in your lifestyle. Here is a brief summary of the steps you must take to make these changes:

1. Define your needs realistically and make an accurate self-assessment.

2. Define your goals. Make them reasonable, but don't be afraid to set challenging objectives.

3. Develop a plan of action. How do you get from where you

are now to your chosen goal in the most efficient and reasonable manner?

4. Don't feel guilty or worry if you backslide a little. Such emotions can retard your progress in changing your lifestyle.

5. Define your anger and locate its source. Figure out where it comes from and where it is *really* directed. Then turn those anger-related problems into challenges.

6. Become your own best friend and always treat yourself in that manner. Be understanding, loving, patient, and helpful to yourself.

7. Anticipate change by evolution, not by revolution. It probably took you many years to get into your present physical and mental condition, so you can't expect to get back into peak condition in a day. Don't put unrealistic pressure on yourself by establishing an unreasonable timetable for reaching your goals. Take your smaller goals one step at a time and flow easily with the changes. Learn from them.

8. As you reach your interim, short-term goals, reward yourself. Take a day off. Buy something you don't really need. See a movie. It shouldn't all be hard work.

Review the section on lifestyle in the Life Management Self-Evaluation Test, which you'll find at the end of this chapter. Think about what you can do to change some of your ways, using suggestions you've just read about. Then set a goal you think you can reach in the next year.

NOW IT'S UP TO YOU

Have you reached out yet and taken a grasp on wellness for yourself?

This book has been an effort to show you how to do that as quickly, effectively, and simply as possible. Accept the challenge. Don't be a spectator in life. Be the best person you can be, the person you were always capable of becoming, the person you were meant to be. You'll feel terrific if you do!

Now, go to the final section of the book to plot your new health goals and to set up your own individual progress chart.

My Lifestyle

Basic information about myself

	Points
I have worked in a smoky office for 16 or more years	− 3
I have worked in a smoky office for 10-15 years	− 2
I have worked in a smoky office for 1-9 years	− 1
I have lived in a smoggy area such as Los Angeles for 10 or more years	− 2
I have lived in a smoggy area such as Los Angeles for 1-9 years	− 1
I have had emphysema (breathing obstruction) for 10 years or more	− 3
I have had emphysema for 1-9 years	− 1
I have had a heart attack or heart disease	−10
I have not had a heart attack or heart disease, but have had heart or chest pain (angina)	− 5
I have or have had diabetes	− 5
I have or have had kidney disorders	− 3
I have or have had thyroid conditions	− 3
I have or have had gout	− 3
I have or have had leg cramps or claudication	− 2

Basic information score _____

Smoking and Pulmonary Status

-15	-10	-8	-5
Over 30 cigarettes per day (or inhale pipe/cigar)	21-30 cigarettes per day	10-20 cigarettes per day	1-9 cigarettes per day

-3	1	2
Over 2 cigarettes per day (or pipe/cigar), but not inhale	20 or more cigarettes per day (or inhaled pipe/cigar), but quit less than 5 years ago	19 or less cigarettes per day, but quit less than 5 years ago

3	5	6	7
20 or more cigarettes per day, but quit 5-10 years ago	19 or less cigarettes per day, but quit 5-10 years ago	20 or more cigarettes per day, but quit over 10 years ago	Never smoked, but lived with tobacco smoker for more than 10 years

8	10	10
Never smoked, but lived with a smoker less than 10 years	5-19 cigarettes per day, but quit over 10 years ago	Never smoked or lived with a smoker

Smoking/pulmonary status score _____

Age

Male

3	0	1	2	3	4	5
72 or over	71–68	67–64	63–61	60–57	56–54	53–49

6	7	8	9	10
48–44	43–40	39–35	34–21	20 or under

Male age score _____

Female

3	2	1	0	2	4
79 or over	78–75	74–70	69–66	65–60	59–54

6	7	8	9	10
53–46	45–38	37–30	29–21	20 or under

Female age score _____

Gender

0	1	2	7	8	9	10
Male, stocky, bald	Male, stocky	Male	Female 55 or over	Female 54–50	Female 49–36	Female 35 or under

Gender score _____

Family history

I have the following number of relatives (parents and grandparents) who had heart disease, stroke, or circulatory disorder which occurred between the indicated ages:

0	1	2	3	5	10
1 or more under age 50	2 or more between 50–60 years	1 between 50–60 years	2 over 60 years	1 over 60 years	None

Family history score _____

My total lifestyle score is _____

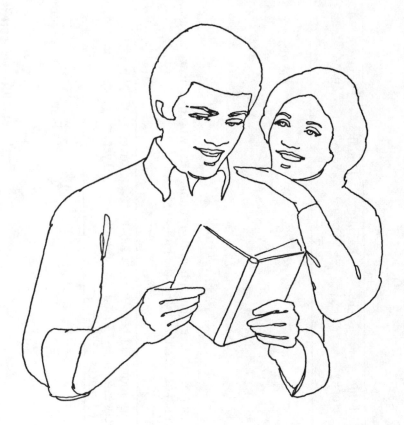

KEEP TRACK OF YOUR PROGRESS TOWARD STAYING WELL THE REST OF YOUR LIFE

Here is how you can use the Life Management Self-Evaluation Test—and a Staying Well scorecard—to help make what you've learned about Staying Well stay with you.

You answered all the questions on the test at the end of Chapter 1 and found out where you stand currently on health and fitness. Then at the end of Chapters 2, 3, 4, and 5, you thought about how much you could do to improve your scores over the next year by setting goals for your diet habits, your exercise program, your efforts to relieve the harmful stresses in your life, and your lifestyle.

Now, on the next page, mark your present position—the score you made when you first took the test. On the Staying Well scorecard, put your score in the appropriate spot on the line at the left-hand side of the scorecard marked "Where You Are Now" (multiple scorecards are included so that you can make this a family program).

Next, add up the scores at the end of Chapters 2, 3, 4, and 5, and put the total score at the right-hand side of the chart, on the line marked "Your Goal."

There are four lines on which to plot your progress after 3 months, 6 months, 9 months, and 12 months. At the end of each time period, retake the Life Management Test (an extra test follows the progress charts), and put your total score on the appropriate line. Then you'll see how you're progressing toward your goal.

Keeping track of yourself on the scorecard will help you see, as well as feel, what your changed lifestyle is doing for your health and fitness. Good luck and good health!

Your Staying Well Scorecard

	Where you are now	3 mo.	6 mo.	9 mo.	12 mo.	Your goal	
Exceptionally low health risk: +120	120					120	Exceptionally low health risk: +120
Very low health risk: 101-120	110					110	Very low health risk: 101-120
Low health risk: 91-100	100					100	Low health risk: 91-100
Satisfactory health risk: 81-90	90					90	Satisfactory health risk: 81-90
Unsatisfactory health risk: 71-80	80					80	Unsatisfactory health risk: 71-80
Poor health risk: 61-70	70					70	Poor health risk: 61-70
Dangerous health risk: 51-60	60					60	Dangerous health risk: 51-60
Extremely dangerous health risk: 50 and below	50					50	Extremely dangerous health risk: 50 and below
	0					0	

Your Staying Well Scorecard

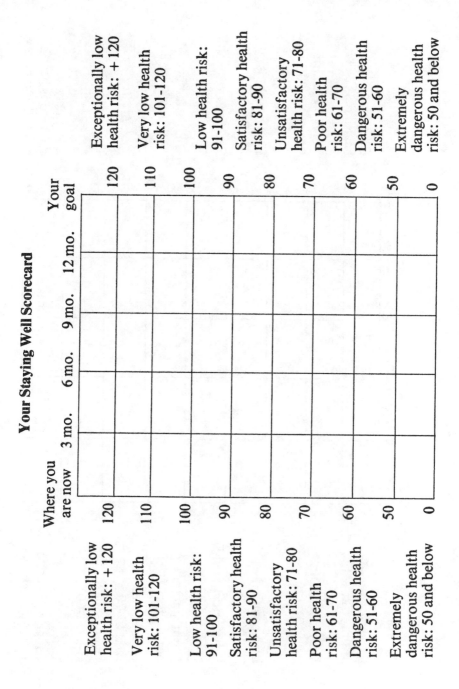

	Where you are now	3 mo.	6 mo.	9 mo.	12 mo.	Your goal	
Exceptionally low health risk: +120	120					120	Exceptionally low health risk: +120
Very low health risk: 101-120	110					110	Very low health risk: 101-120
Low health risk: 91-100	100					100	Low health risk: 91-100
Satisfactory health risk: 81-90	90					90	Satisfactory health risk: 81-90
Unsatisfactory health risk: 71-80	80					80	Unsatisfactory health risk: 71-80
Poor health risk: 61-70	70					70	Poor health risk: 61-70
Dangerous health risk: 51-60	60					60	Dangerous health risk: 51-60
Extremely dangerous health risk: 50 and below	50					50	Dangerous health risk: 51-60
	0					0	Extremely dangerous health risk: 50 and below

Your Staying Well Scorecard

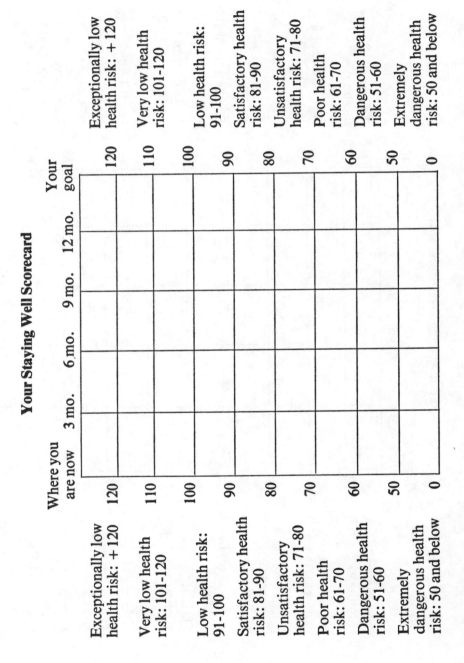

	Where you are now	3 mo.	6 mo.	9 mo.	12 mo.	Your goal	
Exceptionally low health risk: +120	120					120	Exceptionally low health risk: +120
Very low health risk: 101-120	110					110	Very low health risk: 101-120
Low health risk: 91-100	100					100	Low health risk: 91-100
Satisfactory health risk: 81-90	90					90	Satisfactory health risk: 81-90
Unsatisfactory health risk: 71-80	80					80	Unsatisfactory health risk: 71-80
Poor health risk: 61-70	70					70	Poor health risk: 61-70
Dangerous health risk: 51-60	60					60	Dangerous health risk: 51-60
Extremely dangerous health risk: 50 and below	50					50	Extremely dangerous health risk: 50 and below
	0					0	

Your Staying Well Scorecard

	Where you are now	3 mo.	6 mo.	9 mo.	12 mo.	Your goal	
Exceptionally low health risk: +120	120					120	Exceptionally low health risk: +120
Very low health risk: 101-120	110					110	Very low health risk: 101-120
Low health risk: 91-100	100					100	Low health risk: 91-100
Satisfactory health risk: 81-90	90					90	Satisfactory health risk: 81-90
Unsatisfactory health risk: 71-80	80					80	Unsatisfactory health risk: 71-80
Poor health risk: 61-70	70					70	Poor health risk: 61-70
Dangerous health risk: 51-60	60					60	Dangerous health risk: 51-60
Extremely dangerous health risk: 50 and below	50					50	Extremely dangerous health risk: 50 and below
	0					0	

THE LIFE MANAGEMENT SELF-EVALUATION TEST
My Nutrition

	Points
I feel I overeat:	
Usually	0
Occasionally	1
Rarely	3
I have indigestion:	
Often	0
Occasionally	1
Rarely	3
At the table, I salt my food:	
Usually	0
Occasionally	1
Rarely	3
My refined sugar and sweet food consumption is:	
Average or above	0
Less than average	1
Very low	3
My daily sugar substitute servings are:	
Three or more	0
One or two	1
None	3
My daily alcohol consumption is:	
Three or more drinks	0
Two	1
One	2
None	3
My total weekly egg consumption in all food is:	
Ten or more	0
Eight or nine	1
Seven or less	3

	Points
My bread consumption consists of:	
White	0
Light brown/wheat	1
Whole wheat	3
My cereal consumption consists of:	
Boxed cereals, presweetened	0
Vitamin enriched (with extra roughage)	1
Whole grain	3
My daily soft drink (8 oz.) consumption is:	
Three or more	0
One or two	1
None	3
My daily tea consumption is:	
Five or more cups	0
Two to four cups	1
Two cups or less (or herbal tea)	3
My daily coffee consumption is:	
Four or more cups	0
Two or three cups	1
Decaffeinated	2
One cup or less	3
I use:	
Butter	0
Soft or liquid margarine (or none)	3
My daily roughage intake consists of:	
Normal diet	0
Extra salad and raw vegetables	1
Extra source of fiber once or twice a day	3

	Points
Meat in my diet consists mainly of:	
Fatty meats (untrimmed marbled beef, bacon, luncheon meats)	0
Meats (lean beef and pork, veal; chicken, turkey, and fish cooked with skin)	1
Lean meats (fish, chicken, turkey cooked without skin)	3
No meat at all	3
The dairy products in my diet are mostly:	
Whole milk/cream products (include most cheeses) or imitation dairy products or coconut oil	0
Low-fat dairy products	1
Skim milk or no dairy products, low-fat cheeses, low-fat yogurt	3

My nutrition score is _____

My Exercise, Occupation, Recreation, and General Fitness

Activities

	Points
My exercise program consists of:	
Little or no exercise	0
Walking program three or more days per week	1
Easy to moderate exercise three or more days per week	2
Fairly vigorous exercise in exercise attire three or more days per week	5
Heavy exercise in exercise attire three or four days per week	8
Heavy exercise in exercise attire five to seven days per week	10

	Points
My occupational activities consist of:	
Mostly mental activity with little or no manual labor	0
Combination of mental and manual labor	2
Mostly manual labor (I perspire from my work)	4
My recreational activities and hobbies consist of:	
Gardening, doubles tennis, sailing, reading, and other sedentary activities	0
Singles tennis, hiking, light bicycling and other moderately fatiguing activities	2
Prolonged and fatiguing physical activities	4

Activities score _____

Weight

The average person in good physical condition reaches a desirable weight between the ages of 18 and 23. Comparing your weight then and now, you are presently:

10	9	7	5	2	0	-2	-4	-6	-8	-10
At or below that weight	1–3 lbs. over	4–6 over	7–10 over	11–15 over	16–20 over	21–30 over	31–40 over	41–50 over	51–75 over	76 or more over

If you have always been overweight, circle how many pounds overweight you now are.   ·   Weight score _____

Systolic blood pressure

	-5	-3	-2	-1	1	4	6	7	8	9	10
Male	180	160	150	140	135	130	125	121	118	115	110
Female, premenopause	177	157	147	137	132	127	122	119	116	113	108
Female, postmenopause	184	164	154	144	139	134	129	125	122	118	113

If not known, check here _____ and circle 4.   Systolic score _____

Diastolic blood pressure

	-5	-3	-2	-1	1	4	6	7	8	9	10
Male	99	96	93	90	88	84	80	75	70	68	65
Female, premenopause	99	95	90	88	86	83	78	73	68	66	63
Female, postmenopause	99	97	95	92	88	86	82	76	73	68	65

If not known, check here _____ and circle 4.   Diastolic score _____

My total fitness score is _____

My Personality and How I Handle Stress

	Points
I am anxious/nervous:	
Often	0
Occasionally	1
Seldom	3
I would describe myself as:	
Highly competitive	0
Moderately competitive	1
Not competitive	3
When confronted with a situation that bothers or angers me:	
I keep it to myself	0
I may or may not say something	1
I always say something about it	3
Criticism or scolding bothers me:	
Greatly	0
Moderately	1
Hardly at all	3
In my work, success is:	
Very important	0
Moderately important	1
Not important	3
I go out of my way to avoid unpleasant acquaintances:	
Often	0
Occasionally	1
Rarely	3
I have spells of the blues:	
Often	0
Occasionally	1
Rarely	3

	Points
I have disturbed sleep:	
Often	0
Occasionally	1
Rarely	3
People disappoint me:	
Often	0
Occasionally	1
Rarely	3
I am depressed:	
Often	0
Occasionally	1
Rarely	3
In my own work, I am confronted with making important decisions:	
Often	0
Occasionally	1
Seldom	3
"Our country is going to the dogs" is a statement with which I:	
Agree greatly	0
Agree moderately	1
Agree hardly at all	3
I am sexually frustrated:	
Often	0
Occasionally	1
Rarely	3
I am secretive:	
Greatly	0
Moderately	1
Hardly at all	3

My personality/stress score is _____

My Lifestyle

Basic information about myself

	Points
I have worked in a smoky office for 16 or more years	− 3
I have worked in a smoky office for 10-15 years	− 2
I have worked in a smoky office for 1-9 years	− 1
I have lived in a smoggy area such as Los Angeles for 10 or more years	− 2
I have lived in a smoggy area such as Los Angeles for 1-9 years	− 1
I have had emphysema (breathing obstruction) for 10 years or more	− 3
I have had emphysema for 1-9 years	− 1
I have had a heart attack or heart disease	−10
I have not had a heart attack or heart disease, but have had heart or chest pain (angina)	− 5
I have or have had diabetes	− 5
I have or have had kidney disorders	− 3
I have or have had thyroid conditions	− 3
I have or have had gout	− 3
I have or have had leg cramps or claudication	− 2

Basic information score _____

Smoking and Pulmonary Status

−15	−10	−8	−5
Over 30 cigarettes per day (or inhale pipe/cigar)	21–30 cigarettes per day	10–20 cigarettes per day	1–9 cigarettes per day

−3	1	2
Over 2 cigarettes per day (or pipe/cigar), but not inhale	20 or more cigarettes per day (or inhaled pipe/cigar), but quit less than 5 years ago	19 or less cigarettes per day, but quit less than 5 years ago

3	5	6	7
20 or more cigarettes per day, but quit 5–10 years ago	19 or less cigarettes per day, but quit 5–10 years ago	20 or more cigarettes per day, but quit over 10 years ago	Never smoked, but lived with tobacco smoker for more than 10 years

8	10	10
Never smoked, but lived with a smoker less than 10 years	5–19 cigarettes per day, quit over 10 years ago	Never smoked or lived with a smoker

Smoking/pulmonary status score _____

Age

Male

Score	3	0	1	2	3	4	5
Age	72 or over	71–68	67–64	63–61	60–57	56–54	53–49

Score	6	7	8	9	10
Age	48–44	43–40	39–35	34–21	20 or under

Male age score _____

Female

Score	3	2	1	0	2	4
Age	79 or over	78–75	74–70	69–66	65–60	59–54

Score	6	7	8	9	10
Age	53–46	45–38	37–30	29–21	20 or under

Female age score _____

Gender

0	1	2	7	8	9	10
Male, stocky, bald	Male, stocky	Male	Female 55 or over	Female 54–50	Female 49–36	Female 35 or under

Gender score _____

Family history

I have the following number of relatives (parents and grandparents) who had heart disease, stroke, or circulatory disorder which occurred between the indicated ages:

0	1	2	3	5	10
1 or more under age 50	2 or more between 50–60 years	1 between 50–60 years	2 over 60 years	1 over 60 years	None

Family history score _____

My total lifestyle score (six preceding sections) is _____

My total score (nutrition, fitness, personality/stress, and lifestyle) is _____

How Does Your Wellness Add Up?

Extremely dangerous health risk . . . . 50 & below
Dangerous health risk 51–60
Poor health risk 61–70
Unsatisfactory health risk 71–80
Satisfactory health risk 81–90
Very good, low health risk 91–100
Excellent, very low health risk 101–120
Exceptionally low health risk . . . . Over 120

The score you achieve on this test is not a guarantee that you are absolutely a "high" or "low" health risk, since such scores are a result of statistical averages regarding various health risk factors. Your score will, however, give you a good idea of how you compare to others and where you need to concentrate your efforts at improving your health and fitness lifestyle.

Index